IN SEARCH OF EQUITY

Health Needs and the Health Care System

THE HASTINGS CENTER SERIES IN ETHICS

A Continuation Order Plan is available for this series. A continuation order will bring delivery of each new volume immediately upon publication. Volumes are billed only upon actual shipment. For further information please contact the publisher.

IN SEARCH OF EQUITY

Health Needs and the Health Care System

Edited by

Ronald Bayer and
Arthur L. Caplan

The Hastings Center
Institute of Society, Ethics and the Life Sciences
Hastings-on-Hudson, New York

and

Norman Daniels

Tufts University
Medford, Massachusetts

PLENUM PRESS • NEW YORK AND LONDON

Library of Congress Cataloging in Publication Data

Main entry under title:

In search of equity.

(The Hastings Center series in ethics)
Includes bibliographical references and index.
1. Medical ethics. I. Bayer, Ronald. II. Caplan, Arthur L. III. Daniels, Norman,
1942–   . IV. Series. [DNLM: 1. Delivery of health care. 2. Health services
research. 3. Patient advocacy. W 84.1 I35]
R724.I5 1983   174'.2   83-4095
ISBN 0-306-41212-8

© 1983 The Hastings Center
Institute of Society, Ethics and the Life Sciences
360 Broadway
Hastings-on-Hudson, New York 10706

Plenum Press, New York
A Division of Plenum Publishing Corporation
233 Spring Street, New York, N.Y. 10013

Contributors

John Arras, Ph.D., is in the Department of Social Medicine, Montefiore Hospital and Medical Center, Bronx, New York. He also teaches in the Department of Philosophy at the State University of of New York at Purchase, New York, and is currently Visiting Associate Professor of Philosophy at Barnard College, Columbia University. He is the editor of *Ethical Issues in Modern Medicine* (Mayfield).

Jerry Avorn, M.D., is Professor of Social Medicine and Health Policy in the Division on Aging of the Harvard Medical School, Boston, Massachusetts. He is also an Assistant in Medicine at the Beth Israel Hospital, Boston, Massachusetts. He has contributed numerous articles on health policy to such journals as the *New England Journal of Medicine*, the *American Journal of Medicine*, the *Journal of the American Geriatric Society*, and he is on the editorial board of the *Journal of Gerontology*.

Ronald Bayer, Ph.D., is Associate for Policy Studies at The Hastings Center, Institute of Society, Ethics and the Life Sciences, Hastings-on-Hudson, New York. He is the codirector of the Health Policy Research Group at the Center. He is the author of *Homosexuality and American Psychiatry: The Politics of Diagnosis* (Basic).

Arthur L. Caplan, Ph.D., is Associate for the Humanities, The Hastings Center, Institute of Society, Ethics and the Life Sciences, Hastings-on-Hudson, New York. He is the codirector of the Health Policy Research Group at the Center. He recently edited *Concepts of Health and Disease* (Addison-Wesley) with H. Tristram Engelhardt, Jr., and J. J. McCartney.

Norman Daniels, Ph.D., is in the Department of Philosophy at Tufts University, Medford, Massachusetts. He is the author of *Justice and Health Care Delivery* (to be published by Cambridge University Press).

Robert L. Dickman, M.D., is Director of Family Medicine at Mount Sinai Medical Center, Cleveland, Ohio. He has contributed articles on Medical ethics and health policy to the *Journal of Family Practice*, the *Journal of the American Medical Association*, *Journal of Medicine and Philosophy*, among others.

Nancy Neveloff Dubler, J.D., is in the Department of Social Medicine at Montefiore Hospital Medical Center, Bronx, New York. She is the editor of the *Journal of Prison and Jail Health*.

Amy Gutmann, Ph.D., is in the Department of Politics at Princeton University, Princeton, New Jersey. She is the author of *Liberal Equality* (Cambridge University Press).

Mark Siegler, M.D., is in the Department of Medicine, Pritzker School of Medicine, University of Chicago, Chicago, Illinois. He is the author of numerous articles on medical ethics and the philosophy of medicine.

Contents

Introduction

I

Several years ago, when the Carter administration announced
that it would support congressional action to end the public funding of abortions, the President was asked at a press conference
whether he thought that such a policy was unfair; he responded,
"Life is unfair." His remarks provoked a storm of controversy.
For other than those who, for principled reasons, opposed abor-
tion on any grounds, it seemed that the President's comments
were cruel, violating what was thought to be an American commitment to providing equal access to health services to all citizens, regardless of their capacity to pay. Those sentiments had,
in fact, been reflected in public opinion polls that had, for at least
three decades, indicated that Americans supported the proposition that the government should guarantee health care to all.
Ultimately, those beliefs had been translated into the oft-ex-
pressed political demand for a one-class system of health care.[1]
This commitment to equality is rather remarkable. American
society evidences a striking willingness to tolerate vast inequalities with regard to income and wealth. While it guarantees education to all children, there is not even a pretense that the
children of the wealthy and the children of the poor ought to get
precisely the same kind of schooling. While some commitment

[1]Hazel Erskine, "The Polls: Health Insurance," *Public Opinion Quarterly*, XXXIX
(Spring, 1975), 128–143.

has been made to providing publicly supported housing for the poorest, not even the most ardent defenders of such programs argue that public housing should match the housing of the rich or middle-class.

What can account for the special status accorded to health care in the past several decades? It seems clear that at least in part it reflects the belief that an intimate relationship exists between the quality of such care and the quality of life. The fear of disease, suffering, pain, and, ultimately, death provides a common bond cutting across class distinctions. Good health has been considered a primary good and the basis for all other life projects. It is as if good health were a fundamental element in the equality of opportunity so basic to the ideological orientation of Americans. Thus, providing equal access to health services has been perceived not as a matter of providing equal access to the privileges and benefits that generally accrue to the most successful in our society but rather as a fundamental right of citizenship.

Despite the popular appeal of equality in health care, policymakers at the highest levels of government have been less enthusiastic about the development of public programs that would guarantee access to medical care for all Americans. In view of concern about the cost that such programs would entail, limited measures designed to reach specific subgroups in the population have had more appeal. Furthermore, a commitment to incremental shifts in policy have made far-reaching alternatives quite unattractive. Debates within the Carter administration over the desirability of a national health insurance program revealed how difficult the course of reform could be. Now the tone and very content of the official discussion has shifted. Indeed, the next few years may well witness, as a result of the new direction in public welfare policy, a sharpening of inequalities in access to health care. In the era of the expanding welfare state, philosophical inquiries into the problem of justice and health care tended to

have as their main purpose the clarification of the conceptual
foundations for policies designed to reduce the patterns of unequal access to medical services. Such analyses were at times arid
exercises, lacking a firm grasp of the political economy of health
care in America. More frequently they were quite useful, illu-
minating dimensions of public policy in the era marked by official
commitment to the improvement and rationalization of the welfare state. Now that government officials promise a radical rup-
ture with the four-decade course of federal policy, the discussion
of justice in health care will require a confrontation with a changed
political universe. The very discussions that were an integral part
of the reformist ethos of the earlier period will assume a more
critical character.

II

In 1978, under a grant from the Henry J. Kaiser Family
Foundation, the Health Policy Research Group of The Hastings
Center undertook a major study of the ethics of health policy.
The study sought to focus the attention of a broad range of scholars
on the deep and complex problem of fashioning an equitable
health care system. For three years a group of physicians, philosophers, lawyers, health planners, economists, and other social
scientists met to analyze, in a serious and sustained fashion, the
perplexities of health policy.

Among the preeminent tasks the research group set for itself
was a clarification of the goals of the health care system in an era
marked by the extraordinary expansion of the medical domain
and stunning advances in medical technology. Central to that
effort was a confrontation between the views of those who conceive of the goals of medicine in "narrow terms"—the treatment
of disease and the prevention of organic medical problems—and

those who hold a more "expansive" view, one that includes attention to the social and psychological dimensions of health and well-being. Running like a leitmotif through the discussion on this topic and cutting across the two views of the goals of medicine was the attempt to distinguish between health care "needs" and a broader category of health care "wants" or preferences.

Second, the research group paid considerable attention to the increasingly important problem of the relationship between personal behavior and health status. This issue forced the group to confront the terribly difficult question of how society ought to respond to the medical needs of those who have acted in such a way as to "bring upon themselves" the diseases and disabilities that then require the attention of the health care system. From the outset, this issue required an analysis—both empirical and ethical—of the extent to which health-related behaviors could be considered voluntary or primarily the products of various social and psychological factors. Only a resolution of that issue could make possible the appropriate attribution of responsibility and, hence, the development of social policies that could meet the standards of decency and equity.

Third, the group addressed the question of the relationship between experts and lay people in the development of health policy, both at the clinical and social levels. Members of the group undertook analyses of the many ways in which those with a claim to special knowledge and the consumers of health care services have and ought to share responsibility for the making of decisions regarding the allocation of medical care resources to individuals, and to broad segments of the population.

Last, and most important, was the group's investigation of the theme of justice and the health care system. Though originally conceptualized as merely one among the four foci of our work on health policy, it was a concern that ultimately informed our entire project and the consideration of each issue we addressed. Indeed, the question of justice in the allocation of health care resources was so dominant an issue that toward the conclusion of our work all other topics were transformed into subthemes. Thus, whether it was in the discussion of the goals of the health care system, the role of lay people and experts in decision making, or the appropriate response to personal health-related behavior, our focus tended to draw us back to an analysis of how responses to those questions would affect the equity of the health care system.

Although the primary interest of those who worked with the Health Policy Research Group was conceptual, analytic, and prescriptive rather than descriptive, it was always clear that our discussions were rooted in the realities of current allocation of health care services and the prevailing realities of health status in the United States. We were concerned with lacunae in the existing forms of health insurance coverage, the pattern of unequal distribution of health care services, and the differential impact of class, race, and ethnicity on health status. We believed, in short, that a discussion of justice and health care could not, and should not, be abstracted from the very pressing pattern of unmet medical needs in America.

What are those unmet needs? How serious a social problem must be confronted by those who would frame an equitable health care system?

III

Research on the relationship between race, class, poverty, and health status has repeatedly uncovered a stark and disturbing pattern reflecting the impact of social inequality. These findings have underscored the fact that it is not only the level of health care available to the poor but the very conditions of economic deprivation that play a decisive role in determining the health

of the disadvantaged. Here it is only necessary to note the most
salient aspects of the picture.

- In general, infant mortality rates in the United States have
  been declining for all groups over the past decades. In
  1950 it was 29.2 per 1,000 live births; by 1977 it had fallen
  to 14.1 per 1,000 live births. Yet, in this same period, the
  gap between white and black infant mortality rates has
  actually *increased.* In 1950 the black figure was 164% of
  that which prevailed for whites; in 1977 it was nearly
  200%.[2] Thus, in 1977, deaths within the first 28 days after
  birth were 8.7 per 1,000 live births for whites, 14.7 for
  all nonwhites, and 16.1 for blacks.[3]
- The prevalence of many chronic diseases are significantly
  higher than the national average among low-income Americans; the figure for hypertension is 65% higher; for hearing impairments 85% higher; and more than double for
  heart conditions among those between 45 and 64 years of
  age.[4]
- Days of restricted activity reflect the differential impact
  of disease on the poor and on racial minorities. In 1977
  whites averages 17.1 such days per year, while the figure
  for blacks was 21.6. Bed-disability days—a more restrictive category—were 6.6 for whites and 8.9 for blacks.
  When the data are examined by income, there is a striking
  inverse relationship between economic status and disease-
  related restrictions. Those with family incomes of less than

[2]U.S. Department of Health, Education, and Welfare, *Health United States: 1979*
(Washington, D.C.: U.S. Government Printing Office, 1979), p. 11.
[3]Ibid., p. 91.
[4]U.S. Department of Health, Education, and Welfare, *Lead Agency Memorandum on a National Health Insurance Program* (Washington, D.C.: U.S. Government Printing Office, April 3, 1978), p. 6.

$5,000 had 29.6 restricted days of activity; those with $25,000 or more had 12.6 per year.[5]

- These grim facts are reflected in the self-perceptions of the poor and of blacks. When asked to judge their health status, only 10.9% of whites responded "fair" or "poor," while 20.8 of blacks so responded. Those with a yearly income of less than $5,000 responded "fair" or "poor" 24.2% of the time, while those more fortunate—those with $25,000 or more a year yearly income—only responded that way 5.2% of the time.[6]

- Finally, the life-expectancy tables show the ultimate toll of disease and life experiences falling more heavily on nonwhites in America. For whites of both sexes born in 1977, life expectancy was 73.8 years; for nonwhites born in the same year, it was only 64.6.[7]

This pattern for morbidity and mortality has provided the most powerful justification for social policies designed to remove barriers to access to medical care on the part of the poor. Government officials with a commitment to meliorist solutions have preferred to press for the extension of health care services— finding this more compatible with their ideological orientations— rather than to confront the economic and structural roots of disease and ill health. Hence, since the end of World War II, an exceedingly complex array of third-party insurance schemes has emerged to bring necessary health services within the economic grasp of those who had been unable to afford needed care. Health

---

[5]*Health United States*, p. 118. Here it should be noted that there is a complex interaction between poverty and disability. While poverty makes a major contribution to disease, being disabled often results in a significant reduction in personal income and, hence, generates poverty. In the end, of course, the result is the same. Those who are disabled are disproportionately poor.
[6]Ibid , p. 117.
[7]Ibid., p. 90.

insurance became an increasingly important feature of the fringe benefits of the unionized sector of the industrial working class as well as of the salaried middle class. With the enactment of the Medicare and Medicaid programs, insurance was extended to the elderly and the poor. Yet, despite the dramatic extension of such coverage, significant gaps remained. Since coverage to the working population was linked to employment status, the adequacy and existence of medical insurance coverage has been dependent upon the bargaining position of various social strata. Unemployment often brought with it an end to health insurance. The poor who did not fall within the increasingly restrictive definition of "medically needy" also found themselves without protection.

Thus, nearly 24 million Americans have no health insurance.[8] More than 19 million Americans have inadequate insurance that fails to cover basic hospital bills, doctors' services, or medical tests.[9] Some 88 million Americans are inadequately insured against very large medical bills; therefore it is not surprising that in one recent year 7 million families had out-of-pocket medical expenses exceeding 15% of their income.[10]

Despite difficult methodological factors, there is little doubt that substantial gaps remain in the health insurance coverage of the poor and near poor.[11]

The extent to which the officially classed poor and near-poor are excluded from both Medicare and Medicaid, the two major programs designed to guarantee access to health care, varies by state. Overall, *only* 33% of the poor are currently covered by

[8]Joseph A. Califano, "Memorandum for the President: The Basic Decision in Developing a National Health Insurance Plan" (May 22, 1978), mimeo, p. 3.
[9]Ibid.
[10]Joseph A. Califano, "Outline of Briefing, Chart List" (July 29, 1978), mimeo, p. 8.
[11]Karen Davis and Cathy Schoen, *Health and the War on Poverty* (Washington, D.C.: The Brookings Institution, 1978), passim.

Medicaid.[12] In those jurisdictions with relatively enlightened social welfare policies, exclusions are relatively circumscribed: in those where social policy is regressive, the exclusions are striking. A 1975 study notes that in California and New Jersey the exclusions were 6% and 12%, respectively, while the figure for Mississippi was 66% and for Alabama 61%.[13] In Texas, eligibility levels are set so strict that only when family income is at 10% of the poverty level does Medicaid provide coverage not statutorily included under federal law.[14]

Yet, despite these failures, it would be a mistake to ignore the enormous impact Medicare and Medicaid have had in the past decade and a half in reducing the gap between the access to health services enjoyed by the poor and the better off. For example, the proportion of poor children who had not seen a physician for the two years prior to one study had decreased from 33% to 20% in the period between 1964 and 1973.[15] The proportion of low-income women who saw a physician early in pregnancy increased from 58% in 1963 to 71% in 1970.[16] Now some measures show that the frequency of physician contacts among the poor exceeds that among the nonpoor.[17]

When analyzing these data, however, it is crucial to bear in mind that because the poor tend to be sicker than the nonpoor, equality in the frequency of physician visits—to the extent that such visits can be used to measure the meeting of medical needs—

[12]Karen Davis, Marsha Gold, and Diane Makuc, "Access to Health Care for the Poor: Does the Gap Remain?" *Annual Review of Public Health*, 1981, p. 173.

[13]R. J. Blendon, "The Reform of Ambulatory Care: A Financial Paradox," *Medical Care*, XIV(6), 526–34.

[14]Davis, Gold and Makuc, "Access to Health Care," p. 175.

[15]Davis and Schoen, "Health and the War on Poverty," p. 41.

[16]Ibid., p. 43.

[17]Joel C. Kleinman, Marsha Gold, and Diane Makuc, "Use of Ambulatory Medical Care by the Poor: Another Look at Equity," *Medical Care*, XIX (October, 1981), 1014.

is not enough. The poor would need more visits than the better off for medical needs to be met. When examined this way, the advances of the past 18 years become more modest. Thus, in 1976–1978, whites below the age of 17 and below the poverty line whose health status was classified as poor to fair averaged 9.14 physician visits a year, as contrasted with 17.16 visits per year for those whose family incomes was 200% of the poverty level. For blacks, the figures were 5.18 and 10.67 visits, respectively,[18] The difference between poor blacks and relatively advantaged whites was thus almost 260%.

Preventive services continue to reflect important class and ethnic deviations from the standard of equity. Poor women are less likely to receive breast exams, Pap tests, and prenatal care.[19] Because dental services are rarely covered by government programs designed to reach the poor, even the advances witnessed with regard to health services more generally have not been registered in dental care since the enactment of Medicare and medicaid.[20]

Perhaps more disturbing than this pattern of inequality is the fact that the process of reducing the differential between the poor and nonpoor that began in the 1960s may have come to an end. Even before the current assault on social programs began, there were indications that the process of equalization had come to a halt and indeed may have reversed itself.[21] The first indi-

[18]Ibid., p. 1015.

[19]Davis, Gold, and Makuc, "Access to Health Care," pp. 24–27.

[20]*Health United States*, p. 137.

[21]See, for example, Lu Ann Aday and Ronald Anderson, "Equity and Access to Medical Care: A Conceptual and Empirical Overview" (paper presented to the president's Commission for the Study of Ethical Problems in Medicine, Biomedical and Behavioral Research, Washington, D.C., 1981), pp. 23–24.

cations of this change emerged during the Carter years, and they will doubtless become more dramatic in this period of social retrenchment. The federally funded neighborhood health centers that had made an enormous contribution to expanding the access of the poor to health services have been the target of budgetary assault. As cost containment becomes the dominant end of the "supply-side" opponents of social welfare programs, inequality will grow. Those hospitals that are to be closed will be in the inner city and rural areas. Certificate-of-need controls will retard supply expansions where they are needed, as well as in the affluent regions glutted by the presence of physicians and technologically advanced clinical centers.[22]

The efficacy of medical care is not simply a matter of physician contacts but is also dependent upon the organization of the delivery of services. In the early days of the Great Society, it was assumed—or perhaps just hoped—that Medicaid and Medicare would not only increase access to medical treatment but also end the two-class system of care then prevailing. Public assumption of the cost of services would obviate the need for public charity clinics for the poor, thus permitting them to visit private physicians and allowing them to obtain the benefits of an ongoing doctor–patient relationship. The picture today stands in mocking contrast to those assumptions and hopes. A 1978 survey found that 6% of all practicing physicians provided care for one-third of Medicaid patients; over half of Medicaid patients were seen by 16% of physicians.[23] Those physicians with large Medicaid practices were found less likely to be board-certified, were older,

[22]Bruce Vladeck, "Equity Access and the Costs of Health Services" (paper prepared for the President's Commission for the Study of Ethical Problems in Medicine, Biomedical and Behavioral Research, Washington, D.C., 1981), p. 25.
[23]Davis, Gold, and Makuc, "Access to Health Care," p. 23.

and were less frequently affiliated with hospitals.[24] Additionally, the hospital outpatient clinic had emerged as the central element in the provision of medical services to the poor.[25]

In these clinics the poor are likely to be treated by foreign medical graduates and those whose training has yet to be completed.[26] Physician contact tends to be episodic and discontinuous. As a result, drug prescriptions are written by clinicians with less personal knowledge of their patients. Follow-up visits are more likely to be conducted by physicians other than those who made the initial diagnoses.[27]

Finally, the poor are more likely than the nonpoor to be admitted to hospitals as a result of emergency-room contact. When admitted, they tend to be sicker than the more privileged.[28]

IV

The papers collected in this volume, selected from those commissioned by the Health Policy Research Group between 1979 and 1981, address the problems and prospects of transforming the current health care system along more equitable lines. Although the research group was committed to such a change, the papers do not reflect a uniform perspective on the desirability of pursuing particular solutions. Indeed, what will strike the reader

[24]Leon Wyszewianski and Avedis Donabedian, "Equity in the Distribution of Quality of Care" (paper prepared for the President's Commission for the Study of Ethical Problems in Medicine, Biomedical and Behavioral Research, Washington D.C., 1981), p. 18.

[25]Davis, Gold, and Makuc, "Access to Health Care," p. 23.

[26]Vladeck, "Equity Access," p. 13.

[27]Ibid.

[28]Ibid.

is the extent to which very marked disagreements may characterize the discussion among those who have a commitment to
justice in the allocation of health care resources.

Norman Daniels's "Health Care Needs and Distributive Justice" opens the discussion. In this paper, Daniels examines the
claim that health care needs are special, requiring social arrangements that can guarantee access regardless of economic status.
Concluding that such needs are indeed unique because they make
possible the attainment of a "normal range of opportunities" for
all citizens, he recognizes the necessity of drawing a distinction
between those medical interventions that are basic and those that
might more appropriately be considered consumer preferences.
To substantiate the claim that such a distinction can be made,
Daniels relies on an argument that links "needs" to the capacity
for "normal species functioning" while associating preferences
with the broader range of desires involving the enhancement of
life's experiences. Having provided this background and relying
upon John Rawls's theory of justice, Daniels argues that social
institutions ought to guarantee access to a range of services that
can meet health needs. Other mechanisms such as the market
could then be relied upon for the distribution of those health-
related goods and services that are outside the basic range.

For Amy Gutmann, in "For and Against Equal Access to
Health Care," the grounds for extending special recognition to
health care go beyond those of providing the basis for equal
opportunity. For her, working from principles of contemporary
liberalism, there is also a right to relief from pain, as well as a
right to equal respect. It is on this basis that she rests her case
for equal access to health care, recognizing how anomalous that
claim is in an "otherwise inegalitarian society." Unlike Daniels,
Gutmann does not attempt to set limits, by reference to a biological standard, on the range of services to be guaranteed to the
populace; instead, she asserts that such decisions can be made

only through the democratic political process. Thus, there would be for her, as for Daniels, a range of services beyond those governed by the principle of equality. Although she acknowledges the force of the more radical egalitarian proposition that "no health care service shall be available to anyone unless it is available to all," she is willing, for reasons of prudence and principle, to settle for a less extended form of equality in the realm of health care.

From a consideration of macrosocial policy options, Nancy Dubler, in "Jail and Prison Health Care Standards," abruptly shifts our attention to the effort to define medical needs for those subject to prison detention. Studying health care in prisons is an important way of understanding the meaning of basic medical needs. Her choice of the prison is also especially important since, ironically, it is only the prison population that has a judicially defined constitutional right to health care. Using the recent history of court-pressured reform, Dubler provides us with a unique opportunity to observe the interaction of legal judgment, professional medical formulations, and narrow institutional concerns in the fashioning of standards of basic health care. The limitations of that process—its failure to consider seriously the preferences of the prisoners themselves, and its rather unsatisfactory outcomes—suggests to Dubler a lesson for the polity: no process of defining needs that is exclusively professional, that does not consider the preferences of those to be served, can result in adequate care. This is especially so when it is the poor for whom services are being designed. Here she comes close to Gutmann in asserting the importance of the democratic process in policy formulation.

Although much of contemporary discussion regarding the social implications of an expanding medical domain has focused on advances in medical technology, there has been surprisingly little systematic attention to the macro- and microsocial dimensions of the allocations of these new services. That is the task Arthur Caplan has set himself in "How Should Values Count in the Allocation of New Technologies in Health Care?" Using the experience of the U.S. End-Stage Renal Disease Program, he traces the evolution of dialysis from its experimental beginnings to its widespread adoption as a standard form of care. He is thus able to address such issues as: Who ought to bear the burden for developing new technologies? How ought the needs of scientific investigators at the developmental stage be accommodated to the demands of those who believe that their chance for better health or even survival requires access to yet unproven technologies? When the dialysis technology was still new, when machines were few and the demand for them so quickly outstripped availability, there were experiments in microallocation that were socially intolerable. Hence, the assumption by the federal government of the full cost of care for the treatment of end-stage renal disease. That decision, its consequences, and its implications for other advanced medical technologies now being developed make a systematic analysis of the issues raised in Caplan's paper crucial for those concerned with equity in the allocation of health care resources.

The final paper in this volume that deals with the issue of health care as a public policy issue is John Arras's "The Neoconservative Health Strategy." Recognizing that the traditional conservative opposition to government intervention in the structuring of the market for health services can no longer command official support, Arras contends that the neoconservatives have elaborated a series of proposals that would alter the pattern of fee-for-service private practice. For Arras, these efforts reflect the desire to stave off more radical social change in the name of equity. Through a detailed analysis of these proposals, Arras attempts to show that though they entail a superficial willingness to diminish the extent to which inequities characterize the delivery of health care services, they would, in fact, preserve those inequalities. Indeed, he conludes that these neoconservative strategies represent an effort to restructure health care without reforming it on publicly supported egalitarian grounds.

In an effort to underscore the intimate relationship between practices at the micro- and macrosocial levels of health care, the last three contributors to this volume pay close attention to the special character of the clinical relationship in medicine. In "Operationalyzing Respect for Persons," Robert Dickman alerts us to a mistaken premise of so much of the research on the delivery of health care by noting that the quality of such care must be taken into account as well as the ease of access to the units of service. Patients experience their interaction with health care providers as a crucial element in the adequacy of the services they receive. Grim surroundings, so typical of clinical settings for the poor, have a direct impact on their perceptions of medical care. If, as Gutmann argues, equal access is in part founded upon respect for persons, then medical care must reflect that respect. Only by examining the conditions of medical practice can we begin to appreciate this dimension of the search for equity.

In his contribution entitled "Needs, Wants, Demands, and Interests," Jerry Avorn notes that the transformation of medical needs (defined in biological terms) into conscious wants or desires, and then into demands, takes place within the context of the medical relationship. Under what conditions does the appropriate transformation occur, and when is it blocked? Under what conditions do wants and demands reflect something other than baseline needs? Turning from the patient to the physician, Avorn highlights the extent to which the behavior of clinicians often reflects professional needs that are not those of care-seekers. The commitment to research and the pursuit of comprehensive medical knowledge can, in fact, drive the physician to pursue courses of action that the patient may find antagonistic to his or her own medical needs. For Avorn, the attempt to structure a clinical relationship within which the needs of both doctors and patients are given appropriate consideration respresents a central element in the search for an equitable framework for health care.

Finally, Mark Siegler, in "Physicians' Refusals of Patient Demands," addresses a problem that has begun to receive increasing public attention. How ought the clinician respond to the request for care that is deemed inappropriate? In part, this issue has surfaced because third-party reimbursements have ruptured the traditional link between payment and service, thus attenuating the role of financial considerations in patients' decisions to seek medical intervention. But, for Siegler, the problem would present itself even in those cases where the patient assumed the full burden of paying for care considered unnecessary or contraindicated. Physicians as moral agents would still have an obligation to use their professional judgments to limit care to that which seemed medically necessary. Although Siegler asserts that the core of his concern is not macroallocational, it is clear that the willingness of clinicians to refuse inappropriate demands will have a major impact on the viability of any future social arrangement in which basic health care is provided as a matter of social right. Then physicians will serve as gatekeepers protecting public resources from avoidable pressures.

What is the relevance of papers such as these in a period characterized by retrenchment in social programs, a period in which interest at the policymaking level is primarily concerned with the reduction of public expenditures rather than the extension of social benefits to those who are at this point unprotected? Given the outlook for the development of a broad national health insurance program, discussions like those that dominate this volume take on an almost utopian character. But, as Karl Mannheim[29] showed us, utopian thought is crucial to the effort to overcome

[29]Karl Mannheim, *Ideology and Utopia*, (New York: Harcourt Brace Jovanovich, 1955).

the injustices that are masked by all dominant ideologies. Certainly there is a role for such thought in this period. To those stunned by the implications of the current trend in social policy generally and health policy more specifically, the papers assembled in this volume may provide a reflective moral foundation for their critique. Such a moral foundation may serve to illuminate what will certainly be a major and acrimonious public debate in the next years.

RONALD BAYER

Norman Daniels

Health Care Needs and Distributive Justice

Why a Theory of Health Care Needs?

A theory of health care needs should serve two central purposes.
First, it should illuminate the sense in which we—at least many
of us—think health care is "special" and that it should be treated
differently from other social goods. Specifically, even in societies
in which poeple tolerate (and glorify) significant and pervasive
inequalities in the distribution of most social goods, many feel
there are special reasons of justice for distributing health care
more equally. Some societies even have institutions for doing so.
To be sure, others argue it is perverse to single out health care
in this way, or that if we have reasons for doing so, they are

Norman Daniels ● Department of Philosophy, Tufts University, Medford, Massachusetts 02155. Research for this chapter was supported by Grant Number HS03097 from the National Center for Health Services Research, OASH, and by a Tufts Sabbatical Leave. I am also indebted to the Commonwealth Fund, which sponsored a seminar on this material at Brown University. Earlier drafts benefited from presentations to the Hastings Center Institute project on Ethics and Health Policy (funded by the Kaiser Foundation), a NCHSR staff seminar, and colloquia at Tufts, NYU Medical Center, University of Michigan, and University of Georgia. This essay is excerpted from my *Justice and Health Care Delivery*, Cambridge University Press, in preparation.

rooted in charity, not justice. In any case, a theory of health care needs should show their connection to other central notions in an acceptable theory of justice. It should help us see what kind of social good health care is by properly relating it to social goods whose importance is similar and for which we may have a clearer grasp of appropriate distributive principles.

Second, such a theory should provide a basis for distinguishing the more from the less important among the many kinds of things health care does for us. It should tell us which health care services are "more special" than others. Thus, a broad category of health services functions to improve quality of life, not to extend or save it. Some of these services restore or compensate for diminished capacities and functions; others improve life quality in other ways. We do draw distinctions about the urgency and importance of such services. Our theory of health care needs should provide a basis for a reasonable set of such distinctions. If we can assume some scarcity of health care resources,[1] and if we cannot (or should not) rely just on market mechanisms to allocate these resources, then we need such a theory to guide macroallocation decisions about priorities among health care needs.

In short, a theory of health care needs must come to grips with two widely held judgments: that there is something especially important about health care and that some kinds of health care are more important than others. The philosophical task is to assess, explain, and justify or modify these distinctions we make about the importance of different wants, interests, or needs. After considering a preliminary objection to the claim that we need a theory of health care needs, (see pp. 3–5) I shall offer an account of basic needs in general (p. 6–11) and health care needs in particular (p. 12–16). These needs are important to maintaining

---

[1] The objection that health care resources are scarce only because we waste money on frivolous things presupposes distinctions that a theory of needs should illuminate.

normal species functioning, and such normal functioning, in turn, is an important determinant of the range of opportunity open to an individual. This connection to opportunity helps clarify the kind of social good health care is and provides the basis for subsuming health care institutions under principles of distributive justice.

A Preliminary Objection

Before turning to the theory, I would like to address one objection to the project as a whole, for there is reason to think that talk about health care needs and their priorities both is avoidable and undesirable. The objection, which challenges the assumption that we cannot rely on medical markets even where there is adequate income redistribution, can be put as follows: Suppose we could agree on a theory of distributive justice that gives us a notion of *fair income share*. Then individuals could protect themselves against the risk of needing health care by voluntary insurance schemes. Each person would be responsible for buying insurance at the level of protection he or she desired. No one (except children and the congenitally handicapped) would have a *claim* on social resources to meet health care needs unless he or she were prudent enough to buy the relevant insurance (which does not preclude charity). Resource allocation to meet demand, expressed through varying insurance packages, could be accommodated by the medical market provided that appropriate competitive conditions obtained. In this way there would be protection against expensive but rare needs for health care, for which relatively inexpensive insurance could be bought; so too, common but inexpensive services could either be risk-shared through insurance or, if preferred, paid out of pocket without great sacrifice. But expensive and potentially common "needs"—

for example, to be provided with artificial hearts or to be cry-
ogenically preserved—would not become a drain on social resources, since individuals who wanted protection against the risks
of facing such needs would have to buy expensive insurance out
of their own fair shares. This way of meeting health needs would
not create a bottomless pit that would swallow up all available
social resources.[2]

Sometime needs-based theories are criticized because they
give us too small a claim on social resources, providing only a
floor on deprivation.[3] In contrast, the objection we face here
warns against granting precedence to the satisfaction of needs
because we then allow too great a claim on social resources. I
postpone to the end of this essay a consideration of how a need-
based theory can avoid this problem. Similarly, I shall not here
defend the assumption that medical markets fail to be an acceptable allocative mechanism.[4] Instead, I would like to suggest
that the insurance scheme fails to obviate the need for a theory
of health care needs.

---

[2]I paraphrase Charles Fried, *Right and Wrong* (Cambridge, Mass.: Harvard
University Press, 1978), pp. 126ff. See my comments on Fried's proposal in
"Rights to Health Care: Programmatic Worries," *Journal of Medicine and Philosophy*, IV (June, 1979), 174–91. I ignore here an issue of paternalism that
Fried may have wanted to pursue but which is better raised when fair shares
are clearly large enough to purchase a reasonable insurance package. Should the
premium be compulsory?

[3]Needs-based theories cut two ways. Egalitarians use them to criticize the failure
of inegalitarian systems to meet basic human needs. Inegalitarians use them to
justify providing only minimally for basic needs while allowing significant inequalities above the floor. Here I resist the temptation to respond to the inegalitarian by expanding the category of needs to consume such inequalities.

[4]Arrow's classic paper traces the anomalies of the medical market to the uncer-
tainties in it. My analysis has a bearing on the further moral issue of whether
health care ought to be marketed in an ideal market. Cf. Kenneth Arrow, "Uncertainty and the Welfare Economics of Medical Care," *American Economic
Review*, LIII (1963), 941–73.

The key assumption underlying this scheme is that the prudent citizen will be able to buy a *reasonable* health care insurance package from his or her fair share. Such a package can meet the health care needs it is *reasonable for people to want to be protected against*. However, if some fair shares turn out to be inadequate to pay the premium for such a package, then there is something unacceptable about them. Intuitively, they are not fair to those people. But we can describe such a benefit package, and thus determine minimum constraints on a fair share, only if we already use a notion of basic or reasonable health care needs— those that it is rational for a prudent person to insure against. Therefore the "fair share plus insurance" approach only *appears* to avoid talk about health care needs. Either it must smuggle such a theory in when it arrives at constraints on fair shares or else it is open to the objection that the shares are not fair.

There is another way in which a theory of health care needs is implicit in the insurance-scheme market approach: the approach puts health care needs on a par with other wants and preferences and allows them to compete for resources, with no constraints other than market mechanisms operating.[5] But such a stance, far from avoiding the need to develop a theory of needs, already *is* a view of health care needs. It sees them as one kind of preference among many, with no special claim on social resources except that which derives from strength of preference. To be sure, where strength of preference is high, needs may be met; but strength may vary in ways that fail to reflect the importance we ought (and usually do) ascribe to health care. Such a market view needs justification, and it is not a justification simply to point to the *existence* of such a market.

[5]The presence of people with preferences for more-than-reasonable coverage may result in inflationary pressures on the premium for "reasonable" insurance packages. Therefore interference in the market is likely to be necessary to protect the adequacy of fair shares.

Needs and Preference

Not All Preferences Are Created Equal

Before turning to health care needs in particular, it is worth noting that the concept of needs has been in philosophical disrepute, and with some good reason. The concept seems both too weak and too strong to get us very far toward a theory of distributive justice. Too many things become needs, and too few, and finding a middle ground seems to involve many of the issues of distributive justice one might hope to resolve by appeal to a clear notion of needs.

It is easy to see why too many things appear to be needs. Without abuse of language, we refer to the means necessary to reach any of our goals as "needs." To reawaken memories of the neighborhood delicatessen of my childhood, I need only the smell of sour pickles in a barrel. To paint my son's swing set, I need a clean brush. The problem of the importance of needs seems to reduce to the problem of the importance or urgency of preferences or wants in general (leaving aside the fact that not all the things we need are expressed as preferences).[6]

But just as not all preferences are on a par—some are more important than others—so too not all the things we say we need are. It is possible to pick out various things we say we need, including needs for health care, that play a special role in a variety of moral contexts. Taking a cue from T. M. Scanlon's discussion in "Preference and Urgency,"[7] we should distinguish *subjective*

[6]For emphasis, we often refer to things we simply desire or want as things we need. Sometimes we invoke a distinction between noun and verb uses of the word *need* so that not everything we say we need counts as *a need*. Any distinction we might draw between noun and verb uses depends on our purposes and the context and would still have to be explained by the kind of analysis I undertake above.

[7]T. M. Scanlon, "Preference and Urgency," *Journal of Philosophy*, LXXVII (November, 1975), 655–69.

and *objective* criteria of well-being. We need *some* such criterion to assess the importance of competing claims on resources in a variety of moral contexts. A *subjective* criterion uses the relevant individual's own assessment of how well off he or she is with and without the claimed benefit to determine the importance of that person's preference or claim. An *objective* criterion invokes a measure of importance independent of the individual's own assessment, for example, independent of the *strength* of that person's preference.

In contexts of distributive justice and other moral contexts, we do *in fact* appeal to some *objective* criteria of well-being. We refuse to rely solely on subjective ones. If I appeal to my friend's duty of beneficence in requesting $100, I will most likely get quite a different reaction if I tell him I need the money for root-canal surgery, than if I tell him I need the money to go to the Brooklyn neighborhood of my childhood to smell pickles in a barrel. Indeed, it is not likely to matter in his assessment of *obligations* that I strongly *prefer* to go to Brooklyn. Nor is it likely to matter if I insist I feel a great *need* to reawaken memories of my childhood—I am overcome by nostalgia. (He might give me the money for either purpose, but if he gives it so I can smell pickles, we would probably say he is not doing it out of any duty at all—that he feels no obligation.) Similarly, if my appeal were directed to some (even utopian) social welfare agency rather than my friend, it would adopt objective criteria in assessing the importance of the request independent of my own strength of preference.

The issue as Scanlon has drawn it, between subjective and objective standards of well-being, is not just a claim about the *epistemic* status of our criteria of well-being. He is surely right that we do not rely on subjective standards of well-being: we do not just accept an individual's assessment of his or her well-being as the *relevant* measure of that person's well-being in important moral contexts. But the issue here is not just that such a measure is *subjective* and we use an *objective* measure. Nor is the issue that we may be skeptical about the feasibility of developing an objective interpersonal measure of satisfaction, so that we therefore use another measure. Suppose we had an intersubjectively acceptable way of determining individual levels of well-being, where well-being is viewed as the level of satisfaction of the individual's *full range of preferences*. That is, suppose we had some deep social utility function that enabled us to compare different persons' levels of staisfaction, given the full-range of their preferences and the social goods they have available. Such a scale would be the wrong scale to use in a broad range of moral contexts involving justice and the design of social institutions— at least it is not just an improvement on the scale we do in fact use. We would continue to use a far narrower scale of well-being, one that *does not include the full range of kinds of preferences* people have.[8] So the real issue behind Scanlon's insightful discussion is the choice between objective truncated or selective scales of well-being and either objective or subjective *full-range* or "satisfaction" scales of well-being. I shall return shortly to consider why the truncated scale *ought to be* (and not just *is*) the measure used in issues of social justice.

One indication that we appeal to an objective, truncated standard is that I might say the root-canal surgery, but not the smell of pickles in a barrel, is something I *really* need (assuming the dentist is right). It is a *need* and not just a desire. The im-

---

[8]The difference might not be in the *extent* but in the *content* of the scale. An objective full-range satisfaction scale might be constructed so that some categories of key preferences are lexically primary to others; preferences not included on a truncated scale never enter the full-range scale except to break ties among those equally well off on key preferences. Such a scale may avoid my worries, but it needs a rationale for its ranking. The objection raised here to full-range satisfaction measures applies, I believe, with equal force to happiness or enjoyment measures of the sort Richard Bradt defends in *A Theory of the Good and the Right* (Oxford, England: Oxford University Press, 1979), chap. 14.

plication is that some of the things we claim to need fall into special categories which give them a weightier moral claim in contexts involving the distribution of resources (depending, of course, on how well off we already are within those categories of need).[9] Our task is to characterize the relevant categories of needs in a way that *explains* two central properties these special needs have. First, these needs are *objectively ascribable:* we can ascribe them to a person even if he does not realize he has them and even if he denies he has them because his preferences run contrary to the ascribed needs. Second, and of greater interest to us, these needs are *objectively important:* we attach a special weight to claims based on them in a variety of moral contexts, and we do so independently of the weight attached to these and competing claims by the relevant individuals. So our philosophical task is to characterize the class of things we need which has these properties and to do so in such a way that we explain why such importance is attached to them.

Needs and Species-Typical Functioning

One plausible suggestion for distinguishing the relevant needs from all the things we can come to need is David Braybrooke's distinction between "course-of-life needs" and "adventitious needs." *Course-of-life needs* are those needs which people "have all through their lives or at certain stages of life through which all must pass." *Adventitious needs* are the things we need because of the particular contingent projects (which may be long-term ones) on which we embark. Human course-of-life needs would include food, shelter, clothing, exercise, rest, companionship, a mate (in one's prime), and so on. Such needs are not themselves deficiencies, for example, when they are anticipated. But a deficiency

[9]Scanlon, "Preference and Urgency," p. 660.

with respect to them "endangers the normal functioning of the subject of need, *considered as a member of a natural species.*" [10] A related suggestion can be found in McCloskey's discussion of the human and personal needs we appeal to in political argument. He argues that needs "relate to what it would be detrimental to us to lack, *where the detrimental is explained by reference to our natures as men and specific persons.*"[11]

The suggestion here is that the needs that interest us are those things we need in order to achieve or maintain species-typical normal functioning. Do such needs have the two properties noted earlier? Clearly they are objectively ascribable, assuming that we can come up with the appropriate notion of species-typical functioning. (So, incidentally, are adventitious needs, assuming that we can determine the relevant goals by reference to which the adventitious needs become determinate.) Are these needs objectively important in the appropriate way? In a broad range of contexts we do treat them as such—a claim I shall not

[10]David Braybrooke, "Let Needs Diminish That Preferences May Prosper," in *Studies in Moral Philosophy,* American Philosophical Quarterly Monograph Series, No. 1 (Oxford, England: Blackwells, 1968), p. 90 (my emphasis). Personal medical services do not count as course-of-life needs on the criterion that we need them all through our lives or at certain (developmental) stages, but they do count as course-of-life needs in that deficiency with respect to them may endanger normal functioning.

[11]McCloskey, unlike Braybrooke, is committed to distinguishing a narrower noun use of *need* from the verb use. See H. J. McCloskey, "Human Needs, Rights, and Political Values," *American Philosophical Quarterly,* XIII (January, 1976), 2f. (my emphasis). McCloskey's proposal is less clear to me than Braybrooke's; presumably our natures include species-typical functioning but something more as well. Moreover, McCloskey is more insistent than Braybrooke on leaving room for *individual natures,* though Braybrooke at least leaves room for something like this when he refers to the needs that we may have by virtue of individual temperament. The hard problem that faces McCloskey is distinguishing between things we need *to develop our individual natures* and things we come to need in the process of what he calls "self-making," the carrying out of projects one chooses, perhaps in accordance with one's nature but not just be way of developing it.

trouble to argue. What is of interest is to see *why* being in such a need category gives them their special importance.

A tempting first answer might be this: whatever our specific chosen goals or tasks, our ability to achieve them (and consequently our happiness) will be diminished if we fall short of normal species functioning. So, whatever our specific goals, we need these course-of-life needs, and therein lies their objective importance. We need them whatever else we need. For example, it is sometimes said that whatever our chosen goals or tasks, we need our health, and so appropriate health care. But this claim is not, strictly speaking, true. For many of us, some of our goals, perhaps even those we feel most important to us, are not necessarily undermined by failing health or disability. Moreover, we can often adjust our goals—and presumably our levels of satisfaction—to fit better with our dysfunction or disability. Coping in this way does not necessarily diminish happiness or satisfaction in life.

Still, there is a clue here to a more plausible account: impairments of normal species functioning reduce the range of opportunity we have within which to construct life plans and conceptions of the good we have a reasonable expectation of finding satisfying or happiness-producing. Moreover, if people have a high-order interest in preserving the opportunity to revise their conceptions of the good through time, then they will have a pressing interest in maintaining normal species functioning by establishing institutions—such as health care systems—which do just that. So the kinds of needs Braybrooke and McCloskey pick out by reference to normal species functioning are objectively important because they meet this high-order interest people have in maintaining a normal range of opportunities. I shall try to refine this admittedly vague answer, but first I want to characterize health care needs more specifically and show that they fit within this more general framework.

Health Care Needs

Disease and Health

To specify a notion of health care needs, we need clear notions of health and disease. I shall begin with a narrow, if not uncontroversial, "biomedical" model of disease and health. The basic idea is that health is the absence of disease and that diseases (I here include deformities and disabilities that result from trauma) are *deviations from the natural functional organization of a typical member of a species.*[12] The task of characterizing this natural functional organization falls to the biomedical sciences—which must include evolutionary theory, since claims about the design of the species and its fitness to meeting biological goals underlie at least some of the relevant functional ascriptions. The task is the same for man and beast with two complications. For humans we require an account of the species-typical functions that permit us to pursue biological goals as social animals. So there must be a way of characterizing the species-typical apparatus underlying such functions as the acquisition of knowledge, linquistic communication, and social cooperation. Moreover, adding mental disease and health to the picture complicates the issue further, most particularly because we have a less well developed theory of species-typical mental functions and functional organization. The "biomedical" model clearly presupposes that we can, in theory, supply the missing account and that a reasonable part of

---

[12]The account here draws on a fine series of articles by Christopher Boorse; see "On the Distinction Between Disease and Illness," *Philosophy and Public Affairs,* V (Fall, 1975) 49–68; "What a Theory of Mental Health Should Be," *Journal of the Theory of Social Behavior,* VI, no. 1, 61–84; "Health as a Theoretical Concept," *Philosophy of Science,* XL (1977), 542–73. See also Ruth Macklin, "Mental Health and Mental Illness: Some Problems of Definition and Concept Formation," *Philosophy of Science,* XXXIX (September, 1972), 341–65.

what we now take to be psychopathology would show up as diseases.[13]

The biomedical model has two controversial features. First, the deviations that play a role in the definition of disease are from species-typical functional organization. In contrast, some treat health as an idealized level of fully developed functioning, as in the WHO definition.[14] Others insist that the notion of disease is strictly normative and that diseases are deviation from socially preferred functional norms.[15] Still, the WHO definition seems to conflate notions of health with those of general well-being, satisfaction, or happiness, thus overmedicalizing the domain of social philosophy. And historical arguments showing that "deviant" functioning—for example, "Drapetomania" (the running-away disease of slaves) or masturbation—has been medicalized and viewed as disease do not establish the strongly normative thesis that deviance from social norms of functioning constitutes disease. So I shall accept the first feature of the model, noting, of course, that the model does not exclude normative judgments *about* diseases, for example, about which are undesirable or which excuse us from normally criticizable behavior and justify our entering a "sick role." These judgments circumscribe the normative notion of illness or sickness, not the theoretically more basic

[13]Boorse, "What a Theory of Mental Health Should Be," p. 77.

[14]"Health is a state of complete physical, mental and social well-being, and not merely the absence of disease or infirmity." From the Preamble to the Constitution of the World Health Organization. Adopted by the International Health Conference, New York, 19 June–22 July, 1946, signed 22 July, 1946. *Official Record of the World Health Organization*, II, no. 100. See Daniel Callahan, "The WHO Definition of 'Health'," *The Hastings Center Studies*, I (1973), 77–88.

[15]See H. Tristram Engelhardt, Jr., "The Disease of Masturbation: Values and the Concept of Disease," *Bulletin of the History of Medicine*, XLVIII (Summer, 1974), 234–48.

notion of disease (which thus admittedly departs from looser ordinary usage).[16]

Second, pure forms of the biomedical model also involve a deeper claim, namely that species-normal functional organization can itself be characterized without invoking normative or value judgments. Here the debate turns on hard issues in the philosophy of biology.[17] Fortunately, these need not detain us, since my discussion does not turn on so strong a claim. It is enough for my purposes if the line between disease and the absence of disease is, for the general run of cases, *uncontroversial* and ascertainable through publicly acceptable methods—for example, primarily those of the biomedical sciences. It will not matter if there is some relativization of what counts as a disease category to some features of social roles in a given society, and thus to some normative judgments, provided the core of the notion of species-normal functioning is left intact. The model would still, I presume, count infertility as a disease, even though some or many individuals might prefer to be infertile and seek medical treatment to render themselves so. Similarly, unwanted pregnancy is not a disease. Again, dysfunctional noses are diseases, since noses have a normal species function and anatomy. If the dysfunction or deformity is serious, it might warrant treatment as an illness. But deviation of nasal anatomy from individual or social conceptions of beauty does not constitute disease.[18]

[16]Boorse's critique of strongly normative views of disease is persuasive independently of some problematic features of his own account.

[17]For example, we need an account of functional ascriptions in biology. See Boorse, "Wright on Functions," *Philosophical Review,* LXXXV (January, 1976), 70–86. More specifically, we need to be able to distinguish genetic variations from disease, and we must specify the range of environments taken as "natural" for the purpose of revealing dysfunction. The latter is critical to the second feature of the biomedical model: for example, what range of social roles and environments is included in the natural range? If we allow too much of the social environment, then racially discriminatory environments might make being of the "wrong" race a disease; if we allow all socially created environments, then we seem not to be able to call dyslexia a disease (disability).

[18]Anyone who doubts the appropriateness of treating some physiognomic de-

Thus the modified biomedical model still allows me to draw a fairly sharp line between uses of health care services to prevent and treat diseases and uses to meet other social goals. The importance of such other goals may be different and may rest on other bases—for example, in the induced infertility or unwanted pregnancy cases. My intention is to show which principles of justice are relevant to distributing health care services where we can take as fixed, primarily by nature, a generally uncontroversial baseline of species-normal functional organization. If important moral considerations enter at yet another level, to determine what counts as health and what as disease, then the principles I discuss and these others must be reconciled, a task the biomedical model makes unnecessary at this stage and which I want to avoid here in any case. Of course, a complete theory, which I do not pursue, would presumably have to establish priorities among principles governing the meeting of health care needs and principles for using health care services to meet other social or individual goals, such as the termination of unwanted pregnancy or the upgrading of the beauty of the population.[19]

---

formities as serious diseases with strong claims on surgical resources should look at Frances C. MacGreggor's *After Plastic Surgery: Adaptation and Adjustment* (New York: Praeger, 1979). Even where there is no disease or deformity, there is nothing in the analysis I offer that prevents individuals or society from deciding to use health care technology to make physiognomy conform to some standard of beauty. But such uses of health technology will not be justifiable as the fulfillment of health care *needs*.

[19]My account has the following bearing on the debate about Medicaid-funded abortions. Nontherapeutic abortions do not count as health care needs; therefore if Medicaid has as its only fuction the meeting of the health care needs of the poor, we cannot argue for funding the abortions just like any other procedure. Their justifications will be different. But if Medicaid should serve other important goals, like ensuring that poor and well-off women can equally control their bodies, then there is justification for funding abortions. There is also the worry that not funding them will contribute to other health problems induced by illegal abortions.

Although I have deliberately selected a rather narrow model of disease and health, at least by comparison to some fashionable construals, *health care needs* emerge as a broad and diverse set. Health care needs will be those things we need in order to maintain, restore, or provide functional equivalents (where possible) to, normal species functioning. They can be categorized as follows:

1. Adequate nutrition and shelter
2. Sanitary, safe, unpolluted living and working conditions
3. Exercise, rest, and other features of healthy life-styles
4. Preventive, curative, and rehabilitative personal medical services
5. Nonmedical personal (and social) support services.

Of course, we do not tend to think of all these things as included among health care needs, partly because we tend to think narrowly about personal medical services when we think about health care. But the list is not constructed to conform to our ordinary notion of health care; instead, it points out a functional relation between quite diverse goods and services and the various institutions responsible for delivering them.

Disease and Opportunity

The *normal opportunity range* for a given society will be the array of "life plans" reasonable people in it are likely to construct for themselves. The range is thus relative to key features of the society: its stage of historical development, its level of material wealth and technological development, and—even more important—cultural facts about it. Facts about social organization, including the conception of justice regulating its basic institutions, will of course determine how that total normal range is distributed in the population. Nevertheless, that issue of distribution aside, normal species-typical functioning provides us with one clear parameter relevant to defining the normal opportunity range. Consequently, impairment of normal functioning through disease constitutes a fundamental restriction on individual opportunity relative to the normal opportunity range.

There are two important points to note about the normal opportunity range. Obviously, relative to a given range, some diseases constitute more serious curtailments of opportunity than others. But because normal ranges are society-relative, the same disease in two societies may impair opportunity differently; accordingly, its importance may also be assessed differently. Thus the social importance of particular diseases is a notion we plausibly ought to relativize between societies, assuming for the moment that impairment of opportunity is a relevant consideration. Within a society, however, the normal opportunity range abstracts from important individual differences in what might be called *effective opportunity*. From the perspective of an individual with a particular conception of the good (life plan or utility function), one who has developed certain skills and capacities needed to carry our chosen projects, *effective* opportunity range will be a subspace of the normal range. A college teacher whose career and recreational skills rely little on certain kinds of manual dexterity might find his or her effective opportunity diminished little compared to what a skilled laborer might find if disease impaired that dexterity. By appealing to the normal range I abstract from these differences in effective range, just as I avoid appeals directly to a person's conception of the good when I seek a measure for the social importance (for claims of justice) of health care needs.[20]

What emerges here is the suggestion that we use impairment

[20]One issue here is to avoid "hijacking" by past preferences, which themselves define the effective range. Of course, effective range may be important in microallocation decisions.

of the normal opportunity range as a fairly crude measure of the relative importance of health care needs at the macrolevel. In general, it will be more important to prevent, cure, or compensate for those disease conditions that involve a greater curtailment of normal opportunity range. Of course, impairment of normal species functioning has another distinct effect. It can diminish satisfaction or happiness for an individual as judged by that individual's conception of the good. Such effects are important at the microlevel—for example, to individual decision making about health care utilization. But I am here seeking the appropriate framework within which to apply principles of justice to health care at the macrolevel. Therefore we shall have to look further, at considerations that weigh against appeals to satisfaction at the macrolevel.

Toward a Distributive Theory

Satisfaction and Narrower Measures of Well-Being

So far my discussion has been primarily descriptive, not normative. As Scanlon suggests, we do not in fact use a full-range satisfaction criterion of well-being when we assess the importance or urgency of individual claims on our resources. Rather, we treat as important only a narrow range of kinds of preferences. More specifically, preferences that bear on the fulfillment of certain kinds of needs are important components of this truncated scale of well-being. In a broad range of moral contexts, we give precedence to claims based on such needs, including health care needs, over claims based on other kinds of preferences. The Braybrook and McCloskey suggestion gives us a general characterization of this class of needs: deficiency with regard to them threatens normal species-functioning. More specifically, we can characterize health care needs as things we need in order to maintain, restore, or compensate for the loss of normal species-functioning. Since serious impairments of normal functioning diminish our capacities and abilities, they impair individual opportunity range relative to the normal range for our society. If we suppose people have an interest in maintaining a fair and roughly equal opportunity range, we can give at least a plausible *explanation* why they think health care needs are special and important (which is not to say we actually do distribute them accordingly).

In what follows, I shall urge a normative claim: we ought to subsume health care under a principle of justice guaranteeing fair equality of opportunity. Actually, since I cannot here defend such a general principle without going too deeply into the general theory of distributive justice, I shall urge a weaker claim: *if* an acceptable theory of justice includes a principle providing for fair equality of opportunity, then health care institutions should be among those governed by it. Indeed, I shall sketch briefly how one general theory, Rawls's theory of justice as fairness, might be extended in this way to provide a distributive theory for health care. *But my account does not presuppose the acceptability of Rawls's theory.* If some form of rule or ideal code utilitarianism, or if some other theory establishes a fair equality-of-opportunity principle, my account will probably be compatible with it (though some of the argument that follows may not be).

In order to introduce some issues relevant to extending Rawls's theory, I want to consider an issue we have thus far left hanging. *Should* we, for purposes of justice, use the objective, truncated scale of well being we happen to use rather than a full-range satisfaction scale? Clearly, this too is a general question that takes us beyond the scope of this essay. Moreover, it is unlikely that we could establish conclusively a case against the satisfaction scale by considering the health care context alone.

For example, a utilitarian proponent of a satisfaction or enjoyment scale might claim that the general tendencies of different diseases to diminish satisfaction provides, at worst, a rough equivalent to the "impairment of opportunity" criterion I am proposing.[21] Still, it is worth suggesting some of the considerations that weigh against the use of a satisfaction scale.

We can begin by pointing to a special case where our moral judgment would incline us against using a satisfaction scale, namely the case of "social hijacking" by people with expensive tastes.[22] Suppose we judge how well off someone is by reference to the full range of individual preferences in a satisfaction scale. Suppose further that moderate people adjust their tastes and preferences so that they have a reasonable chance of being satisfied with their share of social goods. Other more extravagant people form exotic and expensive tastes, even though they have shares comparable to those of the moderates, and because their preferences are very strong, they are desperately unhappy when these tastes are not satisfied. Assume we can agree intersubjectively that the extravagants are less satisfied. Then if we are interested in maximizing—or even equalizing—satisfaction, extravagants seem to have a greater claim on further distributions of social resources than moderates. But something seems clearly unjust if we deny the moderates equal claims on further distributions just because they have been modest in forming their tastes. With regard to tastes and preferences that *could have been otherwise* had the extravagants chosen differently, it seems reasonable to hold them *responsible* for their own low level of satisfaction.[23]

A more general division of responsibility is suggested by this

[21]Presumably, he must also claim that we improve satisfaction more by treating and preventing disease than by finding ways to encourage people to adjust to their conditions by reordering their preference curves.

[22]I draw on Rawls's "Social Unity and the Primary Goods," in Amartya Sen and Bernard Williams, eds., *Beyond Utilitarianism* (Cambridge, England: Cambridge University Press, 1982).

[23]Here again the utilitarian proponent of the satisfaction scale may issue a typical

hijacking case. Rawls urges that we hold *society* responsible for guaranteeing the individual a fair share of basic liberties, opportunity, and all-purpose means, like income and wealth, needed for pursuing individual conceptions of the good. But the *individual* is responsible for choosing ends in such a way that there is a reasonable chance of satisfying them under such just arrangements.[24] Consequently, the special features of an individual's conception of the good—here extravagant tastes and resulting dissatisfaction—do not give rise to any special claims of justice on social resources. This suggestion about a division of responsibility is really a claim about the *scope* of theories of justice: just arrangements are supposed to guarantee individuals a reasonable share of certain basic social goods that constitute the relevant— truncated—scale of well-being for purposes of justice. The immediate object of justice is not, then, happiness or the satisfaction of desires, although just institutions provide individuals with an acceptable framework within which they can seek happiness and pursue their interests. But individuals remain responsible for the choice of their ends, so there is no injustice in not having sufficient means to reach extravagant ends.

Obviously, a full defense of this claim about the scope of justice and the social division of responsibility, and thus about the reasons for using a truncated scale of well-being, cannot rest on isolated intuitions about cases like the hijacking one. In Rawls's case, a full argument involves the claim that adopting a satisfaction scale commits us to an unacceptable view of persons as mere "containers" for satisfactions, one that departs significantly from

---

promissory note, assuring us that maximizing satisfaction overall requires institutional arrangements that act to minimize social hijacking.

[24]The division presupposes, as Rawls points out in response to Scanlon, that people have the ability and know they have the responsibility to adjust their desires in view of their fair shares of (primary) social goods. See Scanlon, "Preference and Urgency," pp. 665–66.

our moral practice.[25] Because I cannot pursue these issues here, beyond suggesting that there are problems with a satisfaction scale, I am content to show that there is a systematic, plausible alternative to using a satisfaction scale (and ultimately to utilitarianism) the acceptability of which depends on more general issues. Consequently I stick with my weaker, conditional claim above.

Rawls's argument for a truncated scale is, of course, for a specific scale, one composed of his primary social goods. But my talk about a truncated scale has focused on certain basic needs, in particular, things we need so as to maintain species-typical normal functioning. Health care needs are paradigmatic among these. The task that remains is to fit the two scales together. My analysis of the relation between disease and normal opportunity range provides the key to doing that.

Extending Rawls's Theory to Health Care

Rawls's *index of primary social goods*—his truncated scale of well-being used in the contract—includes five types of social goods: (1) a set of basic liberties, (2) freedom of movement and choice of occupation against a background of diverse opportunities, (3) powers and prerogatives of office, (4) income and wealth,

[25]Satisfaction scales leave us no basis for not wanting to *be* whatever person, construed as a set of preferences, has higher satisfaction. To borrow Bernard Williams's term, they leave us with no basis for insisting on the *integrity* of persons. See Rawls, "Social Unity and the Primary Goods." The view that issues here turn in a fundamental way on the nature of persons is pursued in Derek Parfit, "Later Selves and Moral Principles," *Philosophy and Personal Relations,* ed. by Alan Montefiore (London: Routledge & Kegan Paul, 1973), 137–69; Rawls, "Independence of Moral Theory," *Proceedings and Addresses of the American Philosophical Association,* XLVIII (1974–1975), 5–22; and Daniels, "Moral Theory and the Plasticity of Persons," *Monist,* LXII (July, 1979), 265–87.

(5) the social bases of self-respect. Actually, Rawls uses two sim-
plifying assumptions when using the index to assess how well off
representative individuals are. Thus the two principles of justice[26]
require basic structures to maximize the long-term expectations
of the least advantaged, estimated by their income and wealth,
given fixed background institutions that guarantee equal basic
liberties and fair equality of opportunity. More importantly for
our purposes, the theory is *idealized* to apply to individuals who
are "normal, active, and fully cooperating members of society
over the course of a complete life."[27] There is no distributive
theory for health care because no one is sick.

This simplification seems to put Rawls's index at odds with
the thrust of my earlier discussion, for the truncated scale of well-
being we in fact use includes needs for health care. The primary
goods seem to be *too truncated* a scale once we drop the idealizing
assumption. People with equal indexes will not be equally well
off once we allow them to differ in health care needs. Moreover,
we cannot simply dismiss these needs as irrelevant to questions
of justice, as we did certain tastes and preferences. But if we
simply build another entry into the index, we raise special issues
about how to arrive at an approximate weighting of the index
items.[28] Similarly, if we treat health care services as a specially
important primary social good, we abandon the useful generality
of the notion of a primary social good. Moreover, we risk generating a long list of such goods, one to meet each important

[26]See *A Theory of Justice* (Cambridge, Mass.: Harvard University Press, 1971),
p. 302.
[27]Rawls, "Social Unity and the Primary Goods."
[28]Some weighting problems will have to be faced anyway: see my "Rights to
Health Care" for further discussion. Also see Kenneth Arrow, "Some Ordinalist
Utilitarian Notes on Rawl's Theory of Justice,' *Journal of Philosophy*, LXX
(1973), p. 245–63. Also see Joshua Cohen, "Studies in Political Philosophy"
(unpublished Ph.D. thesis, Harvard University, 1978), esp. part III and
appendices.

need.[29] Finally, as I argued earlier in answer to Fried's proposal about insurance schemes, we cannot just finesse the question of whether there are special issues of justice in the distribution of health care by assuming that fair shares of primary goods will be used in part to buy decent health care insurance. A constraint on the adequacy of those shares is that they permit one to buy reasonable pretection, implying that we already know what justice requires by way of reasonable health care.

The most promising strategy for extending Rawls's theory without tampering with useful assumptions about the index of primary goods simply includes health care institutions among the background institutions involved in providing for fair equality of opportunity.[30] Once we note the special connection of normal species functioning to the opportunity range open to an individual, this strategy seems the natural way to extend Rawls's view that *the subjects* of theories of social justice are the *basic institutions* that provide a framework of liberties and opportunities within which individuals can use fair income shares to pursue their own conceptios of the good. Insofar as meeting health care needs has an important effect on the distribution of health and—

[29]Cf. Ronald Greene, "Health Care and Justice in Contract Theory Perspective," in *Ethics & Health Policy*, ed. by Robert Veatch and Roy Branson (Cambridge, Mass.: Ballinger, 1976), pp. 111–26.

[30]The primary social goods themselves remain general and abstract properties of social arrangements—basic liberties, opportunities, and certain all-purpose exchangeable means (income and wealth). We can still simplify matters in using the index by looking solely at income and wealth—assuming a background of equal basic liberties and fair equality of opportunity. Health care is not a primary social good—neither are food, clothing, shelter, or other basic needs. The presumption is that the latter will be adequately provided for from fair shares of income and wealth. The special importance and unequal distribution of health care needs, like educational needs, are acknowledged by their connection to other institutions that provide for equality of opportunity. But opportunity, not health care or education, is the primary social good.

more to the point—on the distribution of opportunity, the health care institutions are plausibly included on the list of basic institutions that should be regulated by a principle of a fair equality of opportunity.[31]

The inclusion of health care institutions among those that are to protect fair equality of opportunity is compatible with the central intuitions behind wanting to guarantee such opportunity in the first place. Rawls is primarily concerned with *the opportunity to pursue careers*—jobs and offices—that have various benefits attached to them. Therefore equality of opportunity is *strategically* important: a person's well being will be measured for the most part by the primary goods that accompany placement in such jobs and offices.[32] Rawls argues that it is not enough to eliminate formal or legal barriers facing those who seek such jobs—for example, barriers based on race, class, ethnic, or sex. Rather, positive steps should be taken to enhance the opportunity of those who are disadvantaged by such social factors as family background.[33] The point is that none of us *deserves* the advantages conferred by accidents of birth, either the genetic or social advantages. These advantages from the "natural lottery" are morally arbitrary, and to let them determine individual opportunity—and reward and success in life—is to confer arbitrariness on the outcomes. Therefore positive steps—for example, through the

[31]Here I shift emphasis from Rawls, when he remarks that health is a *natural* as opposed to *social* primary good because its possession is less influenced by basic institutions. See *A Theory of Justice*, p. 62. Moreover, it seems to follow that where health care is generally inefficacious—say, in earlier centuries—it loses its status as a special concern of justice and the "caring" it offers may more properly be viewed as a concern of charity.

[32]The ways in which disease affects normal opportunity range are more extensive than the ways in which it affects opportunity to pursue careers, a point I return to later.

[33]Of course, the effects of family background cannot all be eliminated. See *A Theory of Justice*, p. 74.

educational system—are to be taken to provide fair equality of opportunity.[34]

But if it is important to use resources to counter the advantages in opportunity that come to some in the natural lottery, it is equally important to use resources to counter the natural disadvantages induced by disease (and since class-differentiated social conditions contribute significantly to the etiology of disease, we are reminded that disease is not just a product of the natural component of the lottery). But this does not mean that we are committed to the futile goal of eliminating all natural differences between persons. Health care has normal functioning as its goal; therefore it concentrates on a specific class of obvious disadvantages and tries to eliminate them. That is its limited contribution to guaranteeing fair equality of opportunity.

The approach taken here allows us to draw some interesting parallels between education and health care, for both are strategically important contributors to fair equality of opportunity. Both address needs that are not equally distributed among individuals. Various social factors—such as race, class, and family background—may produce special learning needs; so too may natural factors, such as the broad class of learning disabilities. To the extent that education is aimed at providing fair equality of opportunity, special provision must be made to meet these special needs. Here educational needs, like health care needs, differ from other basic needs—such as the need for food and clothing—which are more equally distributed between persons. The combination of unequal distribution and the great strategic impor-

[34]Rawls allows individual differences in talents and abilities to remain relevant to issues of job placement, for example, through their effects on productivity. Therefore fair equality of opportunity does not mean that individual differences no longer confer advantages. Advantages are constrained by the difference principle. See my "Merit and Meritocracy," *Philosophy & Public Affairs*, VII (Spring, 1978), 206–23.

tance of the opportunity to obtain both health care and education puts these needs in a separate category from those basic needs we can expect people to purchase from their fair income shares.

It is worth noting another point of fit between my analysis and Rawls's theory. In Rawls's contract situation, a "thick" veil of ignorance is imposed on contractors choosing basic principles of justice: they do not know their abilities, talents, place in society, or historical period. In selecting principles to govern health care resource-allocation decisions, we need a thinner veil, for we must know about some features of the society, for example, its resource limitations. Still, using the normal opportunity range and not just the effective range as the baseline has the effect of imposing a plausibly thinned veil. It reflects basic facts about the society but keeps facts about individuals' particular ends from unduly influencing social decisions. Ultimately, defense of a veil depends on the theory of the person underlying the account. The intuition here is that people are not defined by a particular set of interests but are free to revise their life plans. Consequently, they have an interest in maintaining conditions under which they can revise such plans, which makes the normal range a plausible reference point.

Subsuming health care institutions under the opportunity principle can be viewed as a way of keeping the system as close as possible to the original idealization under which Rawl's theory was constructed, namely, that we are concerned with normal, fully functioning people with a complete life span. An important set of institutions can thus be viewed as a first defense of the idealization: they act to minimize the likelihood of departures from the normality assumption. Included here are institutions which provide for public health, environmental cleanliness, preventive personal medical services, occupational health and safety, food and drug protection, nutritional education, and educational and incentive measures to promote individual responsibility for

healthy life-styles. A second layer of institutions corrects departures from the idealization. It includes those delivering personal
medical and rehabilitative services that restore normal functioning. A third layer attempts, where feasible, to maintain people
in a way that is as close as possible to the idealization. Institutions
involved with more extended medical and social support services
for the moderately chronically ill and disabled and the frail elderly
would fit here. Finally, a fourth layer involves health care and
related social services for those who can in no way be brought
closer to idealization. Terminal care and care for the seriously
mentally and physically disabled fit here, but they raise serious
issues which may not be simple issues of justice. Indeed, by the
time we get to the fourth layer, moral virtues other than justice
become prominent.

Worries and Qualifications

I would like to address two kinds of worries that arise in
response to the approach of equality of opportunity that I have
been sketching, although no doubt there are others.[35] One is that
the account cannot be *exhaustive* of distributive issues in health

[35]For example, appeals to equality of opportunity have historically played a conservative, deceptive role, blinding people to the injustice of class and race
inequalities in rewards. Historically, appeals to the ideal of equal opportunity
have implicitly justified strongly competitive individual relations. More con-
cretely, we often find institutions, like the U.S. educational system, praised as
embodying (at least approximately) that ideal, whereas there is strong evidence
that the system function primarily to replicate class inequalities. See my "IQ,
Heritability and Human Nature" in *Proceedings of the Philosophy of Science
Association, 1974*, ed. by R. S. Cohen (Dordrecht, Netherlands: Reidel, 1976),
pp. 143–80; and (with J. Cronin, A. Krock, and R. Webber) "Race, Class and
Intelligence: A Critical Look at the IQ Controversy," *International Journal of
Mental Health*, III, no. 4, 46–123; and S. Bowles and H. Gintin, *Schooling and
Capitalist America* (New York: Basic Books, 1976).

care—the connection to opportunity is but one consideration among many. A second worry is that the appeal to opportunity is not a *usable* one—it commits us to too much or fails to tell us what we are committed to. Both worries emphasize the degree to which my account is programmatic.

One way to put the first worry is that my account makes the "specialness" of health care rest on quite abstract considerations. After all, when we reflect on the importance of health care needs, many other factors than their effects on opportunity come to mind. Some might say that health care, in a direct and simple way, reduces pain and suffering—and no fancy analysis of opportunity is needed to show why people value this outcome. Still, much health care affects quality of life in other ways, so the benefit of reducing pain and suffering is not general enough for our purposes. Moreover, some suffering, for example, some emotional suffering, though a cause for concern, does not obviously become a concern of justice. Others may point to psychological or cultural bases for our view of health care as special; for example, disease reminds us of the fragility of life and the limits of human existence. But even if this point is relevant to sociological or psychological explanations of the importance some of us attribute to some kinds of health care, I have been attempting a different kind of analysis, one that can be used to justify and not just explain the importance attached to health care. So I have abstracted a central *function* of health care, the maintenance of species-typical functioning, and noted its central *effect* on opportunity. As a result, we are in a better position to frame distributive principles that account for the special way we treat health care, because we can now say what kind of a social good health care is—namely, one that maintains normal opportunity range. My analysis, while not exhaustive, focuses on that general benefit which is most relevant from the point of view of distributive justice.

Still, this qualification does not settle the first worry, which

can be raised in another way. Within the confines of Rawls's theory, fair equality of opportunity, and Rawls's principle guaranteeing it, is concerned solely with access to jobs and offices. In
contrast, my notion of normal opportunity range is far broader.
To be sure, the narrower notion, whatever its problems, is far
clearer than the broader one. But if we stick with the narrower
one, we immediately import a strong age bias into our distributive
theory. The opportunity of the elderly to enter jobs or offices is
not impaired by disease since they are beyond, as the crass phrase
goes, their "productive" years. Thus fair equality of opportunity
narrowly construed seems open to one of the standard objections
raised against productivity measures of the value of life.[36]

There are two ways to respond to this problem while still
adhering to the narrower construal of opportunity. One is to admit
that equality of opportunity is only one among several considerations that bear on the justice of health care distribution. Still,
even on this view, it is an important consideration with broad
implications for health care delivery. A fleshing out of this response would require showing how the opportunity principle fits
with these other considerations. A stronger response is to claim
that the domain of basic considerations of *justice* regarding health
care is exhausted by the equal opportunity principle. Other moral
considerations may bear on distribution, but claims of justice will
be based on the narrowly construed opportunity principle. This
response bites the bullet about the age effect.

If we turn to the broader construal of equality of opportunity,
using the notion of normal opportunity range, the problem reemerges, as do the weaker and stronger responses, but there may

[36]See E. J. Mishan, "Evaluation of Life and Limb: A Theoretical Approach,"
Journal of Political Economy, LXXIX, no. 4 (1971), 687–705; Jan Paul Acton,
"Measuring the Monetary Value of Life Saving Programs," *Law and Contem-
porary Problems*, XL (Autumn, 1976), 46–72; Michael Bayles, "The Price of
Life," *Ethics*, LXXXIX (October, 1978), 20–34.

be more flexibility. The problem reemerges because it might seem that the young will always suffer greater impairment of opportunity than the elderly if health care needs are not met. But a further alternative suggests itself: it may be possible to make the normal opportunity range relative to age. On this view, there is a normal opportunity range for each age (stage of life), but it reflects basic facts about the life cycle and a society's responses to it. Consequently, diseases may have different effects on the young and elderly and their importance will be assessed differently.[37] This approach may avoid the most serious objections about age bias, but it still leaves open the weak claim that it circumscribes the scope of basic claims of justice. The stronger claim may seem more plausible, since the opportunity principle has broader scope on this construal. But employing the broader construal brings with it other serious problems: do arguments that establish the priority of fair equality of opportunity on the narrow construal, with its competitive aspect, extend to the broader notion? These issues and alternatives require more careful discussion than they can be given here.

The second worry, about what commitments the appeal to equal opportunity generates, also has several sources. Certain "hard" cases raise the issue sharply. What does asking for the restoration of normal opportunity range mean for the terminally ill, on whom we lavish exotic life-prolonging technology, or for the severely mentally retarded? We are not required to pour all our resources into the worst cases, for that would undermine our

[37] It would be interesting to know whether this age-relativized opportunity range yields results similar to that achieved by the Rawlsian device of a veil. If people who do not know their age are asked to design a system of health care delivery for the society they will be in, they would presumably budget their resources in a fashion that takes the special features of each stage of the life cycle into account and gives each stage a reasonable claim on resources. Cf. my "Am I My Parents' Keeper?" *Midwest Studies in Philosophy*, VII (1982), pp. 517–540.

ability to protect the opportunity of many others. But I am not sure what the approach requires here, if it delivers an answer at all. Similarly, the approach provides little help with another sort of hard case, the resource-allocation decisions in which we must choose between services that remove serious impairments of opportunity for a few people and those that remove significant but less serious impairments from many. But these shortcomings are not special to the approach I sketch: distributive theories generally founder on such cases. It seems reasonable to test my approach first in the cases where we have a better understanding what kind of health care is owed. In any case, I do not rule out here the strong response sketched earlier to the worry about exhaustiveness—namely, that our problem with at least the first kind of hard case derives from the fact that it takes us beyond the domain of justice into other considerations of right.

The second worry also has more fundamental sources. Suppose supplying a car to everyone who cannot afford one would do more to remove individual impairments of normal opportunity range than supplying certain health care services to those who need them. Does the opportunity approach commit us now to supplying cars instead of treatments?[38] The example is an instance of a far more general problem, namely, that socioeconomic (and other) inequalities affect opportunity (broadly or narrowly construed), not just the health care and educational needs we have picked out as strategically important. But my approach does not require me to deny that certain inequalities in wealth and income may conflict with fair equality of opportunity and that guaranteeing fair equality of opportunity may thus constrain acceptable inequalities in these goods. Rather, my approach rests on the

---

[38]Using medical technology to enhance normal capacities of functions—say strength or vision—makes the problem easier: the burden of proof is on proposals that give priority to altering the normal opportunity range rather than protecting individuals whose normal range is comprises.

calculation that certain institutions meed needs that quite generally have a central impact on opportunity range and which should therefore be governed directly by the opportunity principle.

Finally, the second worry can be traced to the fear that health care needs are so *expansive* (and expensive), given the advance of technology, that they create a bottomless pit. Fried, for example, argues that recognizing claims of individual right to the satisfaction of health care needs would force society to forgo realizing other social goals. He cautions that we would end up worshiping the opportunity to pursue our goals but having to forgo the pursuit. Here we have the other form of the social hijacking argument, hijacking by needs rather than preferences.[39]

Two points can be offered in response to Fried's version of the second worry. First, the narrow model of health care needs that I have given excludes some of the kinds of cases Fried uses to demonstrate the threat of the bottomless pit. Thus Fried's example of retarding the effects of normal aging does not emerge as a *need* on my analysis, since normal aging does not involve a departure from normal species functioning. Such uses of health care technology may be thought important in a particular society. Then, arguments about the relative merits of this use of scarce resources may be advanced. But such arguments would not rest on claims about basic health care needs and thus may have different justificatory force. Still, technology does expand the ways we have (and the costs) of meeting genuine health care needs. So my account of needs at best reduces but does not eliminate Fried's worry.

Second, there is a difference between Fried's account of individual rights and entitlements and the one I am assuming here (which is quite Rawlsian). Fried is worried that if we posit

---

[39]See Fried, *Right and Wrong*, chap. 5. The problem also worries Braybrooke, "Let Needs Diminish."

a fundamental individual right to have needs satisfied, no other social goals will be able to override the claims to all health care needs.[40] But no such fundamental right is *directly* posited on the view I have sketched. Rather, the particular rights and entitlements of individuals to have certain needs met are specified only *indirectly*, as a result of the basic health care institutions acting in accord with the general principle governing opportunity. Deciding which needs are to be met and what resources are to be devoted to doing so requires careful moral judgment. The various institutions which affect opportunity must be weighed against each other. Similarly, the resources required to provide for fair equality of opportunity must be weighed against what is needed to provide for other important social institutions. Clearly, health care institutions capable of protecting opportunity can be maintained only in societies whose productive capabilities they do not undermine. The bugaboo of the bottomless pit is less threatening in the context of such a theory. The price paid is that we are less clear—in general and abstracting from the application of the theory to a given society—about just what the individual claim comes to. The price is worth paying.

These worries emphasize the sense in which my account is sketchy and progammatic. It is worthwhile to reassert that my account is incomplete in other ways as well. I have not argued that opportunity-based considerations are the only ones that should bear on the design of health care systems. Other important social goals—some protected by claims of right or other claims of need— may require the use of health care technology. I have not considered when, if ever, these needs or rights take precedence over other wants and preferences or over some health care needs.[41] Similarly, there is the question whether the demand for equality

---

[40]It is not clear to me how much Fried's side-constraints resemble Nozick's.
[41]See footnote 19 above.

in health care extends beyond some decent adequate minimum—
which we may suppose is defined by reference to fair equality of
opportunity. Should those health care services not considered
basic be allowed to operate on a market basis? Should we insist
on equality even here? These issues are not addressed by my
analysis.[42]

Finally, my account is incomplete because I have concen-
trated on social obligations to maintain and restore health and
have ignored individual responsibility to do so. But there is substantial evidence that individuals can do much to avoid incurring
risks to their health—by avoiding smoking, excess alcohol, and
certain foods and by getting adequate exercise and rest. Now,
nothing in my approach is incompatible with encouraging people
to adopt healthy life-styles. The harder issue, however, is deciding how to distribute the burdens that result when people "voluntarily" incur extra risks and swell the costs of health care by
doing so (by over 10 percent, on some estimates). After all, the
consequences of such behavior cannot be easily dismissed as the
arbitrary outcome of the natural lottery. Should smokers be forced
to pay higher insurance premiums or special health care taxes?
I do not believe my account forces us to ignore the source of
health care risks in assigning such burdens. But at this point little
more can be said because much here depends on very specific
details of social history. In the United States, government subsidies of the tobacco industry, the legality of cigarette advertising,
the legality of smoking in public places, and special subcultural
pressures on key groups (for example, teenagers) all undermine

---

[42]Except where conditions of extensive scarcity leave basic health care needs
unmet, so that there is no room for less important uses of health care services,
or where the existence of a market-based health care system threatens the ability
of the basic system to deliver its important product. Cf. my "Equity of Access
to Health Care: Some Conceptual and Ethical Issues," Milbank Memorial Fund
Quarterly/Health and Society, Vol. 60, no. 1 (1982), pp. 51–81.

the view that we have clear-cut cases of informed, individual decision making for which individuals must be held fully accountable.

Applications

The account of health care needs sketched here has a number of implications of interest to health care planners. Here I can only note some of them and set aside the many difficulties that are encountered in attempting to draw implications from ideal theory for nonideal settings.[43]

Access

My account is compatible with (but does not imply) a multitiered health care system. The basic tier would include health care services that meet important health care needs, defined by reference to their effects on opportunity. Other tiers would include services that meet less important health care needs or other preferences. However the upper tiers are to be financed—through cost sharing, at full price, or at "zero" price[44]—there should be no obstacles (financial, racial, sexual, or geographical) to *initial access* to the system as a whole.

[43]I discuss these difficulties in "Conflicting Objectives and the Priorities Problem," *Income Support: Conceptual and Policy Issues* ed. by Peter G. Brown, Conrad Johnson, and Paul Vernier (Totowa, N.J.: Rowman and Littlefield, 1981), pp. 147–64. My *Justice and Health Care Delivery* develops some applications in detail.

[44]The strongest objections to such mixed systems is that the upper tier competes for resources with the lower tiers. See Claudine McCreadie, "Rawlsian Justice and the Financing of the National Health Service," *Journal of Social Policy*, V, no. 2 (1976), 113–31.

The equality of initial access derives from basic facts about the sociology and epistemology of the determination of health care needs.[45] The "felt needs" of patients are initial though unreliable indicators of real health care needs. Financial and geographical barriers to initial access—say to primary care—compel people to make their own determinations of the importance of their symptoms. Of course, every system requires some patient self-assessment, but financial and geographical barriers impose different burdens in such assessment on particular groups. Indeed, where sociological barriers to the utilization of services exist, positive steps are needed (in the schools, at work, in neighborhoods) to make sure that unmet needs are detected.

It is sometimes argued that problems of access derive from geographical barriers and the maldistribution of physicians within specialties. In the United States, it is often argued that the achievement of a more equitable distribution of health care providers would unduly constrain physicians liberties. It is important to see that no fundamental liberties need be violated. Suppose that the basic tier of a health care system were redistributively financed through a national health insurance scheme that eliminated financial barriers, that no alternative insurance for the basic tier were allowed, and that there were central planning of resource allocation to guarantee the meeting of needs. To achieve a more equitable distribution of physicians, planners would *license those eligible for reimbursement* in a given health planning region according to some reasonable formula involving physician–patient ratios.[46] Additional providers might practice in an area,

[45]See Avedis Donabedian, *Aspects of Medical Care Administration* (Cambridge, Mass.: Harvard University Press, 1973).

[46]I ignore the crudeness of such measures. For fuller discussion of these manpower distribution issues, see my "What Is the Obligation of the Medical Profession in the Distribution of Health Care?" *Social Science and Medicine*, Vol. 15F, no. 4 (December, 1981), pp. 129–133.

but they would be without benefit of third-party payments for all services in the basic tier (or for other tiers if the national insurance scheme were more comprehensive). Most providers would follow the reimbursement dollar and practice where they were most needed.

Far from violating basic liberties, this scheme merely puts physicians in the same relation to market constraints on job availability that face most other workers and professionals. A college professor cannot simply decide that there are people to be taught in Scarsdale or Chevy Chase or Shaker Heights; he or she must accept what jobs are available within universities, wherever they are. Of course, the professor is "free" to ignore the market, but then he or she may not be able to teach. Similarly, managers and many types of workers face the need to locate themselves where there is a need for their skills. So the physician's sacrifice of liberty under the scheme (or variants on it, including a National Health Service) is merely the imposition of a burden already faced by much of the working population. Indeed, the scheme does not change in principle the forces that already motivate physicians; it merely shifts the areas where it is profitable for some physicians to practice. The appearance that there is an enshrined liberty under attack is the legacy of a historical accident, one more visible in the United States than elsewhere, namely that physicians have been more independent of institutional settings for the delivery of their skills than many other workers and even than physicians in other countries. But this too shall pass.

Resource Allocation

My account of health-care needs and their connection to fair equality of opportunity has a number of implications for resource-allocation issues. I have already noted that we get an important distinction between the use of health care services to meet health care needs and their use to meet other wants and preferences. The tie of health care needs to opportunity makes the former use special and important in a way not true of the latter. Moreover, we get a crude criterion—impact on normal opportunity range— for distinguishing the importance of different health care needs, though I have also noted how far short this falls of being a solution to many hard allocation questions. Three further implications are worth noting here.

There has been much debate about whether the U. S. health care system overemphasizes acute therapeutic services as opposed to preventive and public health measures. Sometimes the argument focuses on the relative efficacy and cost of preventive as opposed to acute services. My account suggests that there is also an important issue of distributive justice here. Suppose a system were heavily weighted toward acute interventions yet provided equal access to its services. Thus anyone with severe respiratory ailments—black lung, asbestosis, emphysema, and so on—would be given adequate and comprehensive services as needed. Would the system meet the demands of equity? Not if they were determined by the approach of fair equality of opportunity. The point is that people are differentially at risk of contracting such diseases because of work and living conditions. Efficacy aside, preventive measures have distributive implications distinct from those of acute measures. The opportunity approach requires that we attend to both.

My account points to another allocational inequity. One important function of health care services, here personal medical services, is to restore handicapping dysfunctions, of vision or mobility for example. The medical goal is to cure the diseased organ or limb where possible. Where cure is impossible, we try to make function as normal as possible—through, for example, corrective lenses or prostheses and rehabilitative therapy. But where restoration of function is beyond the ability of medicine per se, we begin to enter another area of services, nonmedical social support (we move from item 4 to item 5 in the list of health care needs presented earlier). Such support services provide the blind person with the closest available functional equivalent of vision; for example, he or she is taught how to navigate, provided with a seeing-eye dog, taught braille, and so on. From the point of view of their impact on opportunity, medical services and social support services that meet health care needs have the same rationale and are equally important. Yet, for various reasons probably having to do with the profitability and glamor of personal medical services and careers in them as compared to services for the handicapped, our society has taken only slow and halting steps to meet the health care needs of those with permanent disabilities. These are matters of justice, not charity; we are not facing conditions of scarcity so severe that these steps to provide equality of opportunity must be forgone in favor of more pressing needs. The point also has implications for the problems of long-term care for the frail elderly, but I cannot develop them here.

A final implication of the account raises a different set if issues, namely, how to reconcile the demands of justice with certain traditional views of physicians' obligations to their patients. The traditional view is that the physician's direct responsibility is to the well-being of patients, that (with their consent) he or she is to do everything possible to preserve their lives and well-being. One effect of leaving all resource-allocation decisions, in this way, to the microlevel decisions of physicians and patients, especially where third-party payment schemes mean little or no rationing by price, is that cost-ineffective utilization results. In the current cost-conscious climate, there is pressure to make physicians see themselves as responsible for introducing economic considerations into their utilization decisions. But the issue raised here goes beyond cost-effectiveness. My account suggests that there are important resource-allocation priorities that derive from considerations of justice. In a context of moderate scarcity, this suggests that it is not possible for physicians to see as their ideal, regardless of cost, the maximization of the quality of care they deliver; pursuing that ideal upsets resource-allocation priorities determined by the opportunity principle. Considerations of justice challenge the traditional (perhaps mythical) view that physicians can act as the unrestrained agents of their patients. The remaining task, which I pursue elsewhere, is to show at what level the constraints should be imposed so as to disturb as little as possible that which is valuable about the traditional view of physician responsibility.[47]

These remarks on applications are frustratingly brief; a fuller development is required if we are to assess the practical import of the account I offer. Nevertheless, I think the account offers enough that it is attractive at the theoretical level to warrant further development of its practical implications.

ACKNOWLEDGMENTS

Helpful comments for this chapter were provided by Ronald Bayer, Hugo Bedau, Richard Brandt, Dan Brock, Arthur Caplan, Josh Cohen, Allan Gibbard, Ruth Macklin, Carola Mone, John Rawls, Daniel Wikler, and the editors of *Philosophy & Public Affairs*.

[47]See Avedis Donabedian, "The Quality of Medical Care: A Concept in Search of a Definition," *Journal of Family Practice*, IX, no. 2 (1979), 227–84; and Daniels, "Cost-Effectiveness and Patient Welfare," *Ethics, Humanism and Medicine*, ed. by Marc Basson (New York: Liss, 1981), 159–71.

2

Amy Gutmann

For and Against Equal Access to Health Care

There is a fairly widespread consensus among empirical analysts that access to health care in this country has become more equal in the last quarter century. Agreement tends to end here, and debate ensues as to whether this trend will or should persist. But before debating these questions, we ought to have a clear idea of what equal access to health care means. Since we cannot define equality of access to health care in a morally neutral way, we must choose a definition that is morally loaded with a set of values.[1] The definition offered here is by no means the only one possible. It has, however, the advantage not only of clarity but

This chapter is a slightly revised version of an essay that originally appeared in *The Milbank Quarterly*.

[1]Norman Daniels, "Equity of Access to Health Care: Some Conceptual and Ethical Issues" (paper presented to The President's Commission for the Study of Ethical Issues in Medicine and Biomedical and Behavioral Research, Washington, D.C., 1981).

Amy Gutmann ● Department of Politics, Princeton University, Princeton, New Jersey 08544. This chapter was prepared under special commission for the President's Commission for the Study of Ethical Issues in Medicine and Biomedical and Behavioral Research and was also sponsored in part by the Hasting Center project on Justice and Health Care funded by the Kaiser Foundation.

also of embedding within it strong and commonly accepted liberal egalitarian values. The debate is better focused upon arguments for and against a strong *principle* of equal access than on disputes over definitions, which tend to hide fundamental value disagreements instead of making them explicit.

An equal-access principle, clearly stated and understood, can serve at best as an ideal toward which a society committed to equality of opportunity and equal respect for persons can strive. It does not provide a blueprint for social change but only a moral standard by which to judge marginal changes in our present institutions of health care.

My purpose in this essay is not only to evaluate the strongest criticisms addressed to the principle—ranging from libertarian arguments for more market freedom to other arguments supporting a more egalitarian principle of health care—but also to examine the sorts of theoretical and practical problems that arise when one tries to defend an egalitarian principle directed at a particular set of institutions within an otherwise inegalitarian society. Since it is extremely unlikely that such a society will be transformed all at once into an egalitarian one, there ought to be room within political and philosophical argument for reasoned consideration and advocacy of "partial" distributive justice—that is, of principles that are directed only to a particular set of social institutions and whose implementation is not likely to create complete justice even within those institutions.

The Principle Defined

A principle of equal access to health care demands that every person who shares the same type and degree of health need be given an equally effective chance of receiving appropriate treatment of equal quality so long as that treatment is available to anyone. Stated in this way, the equal access principle does not establish whether a society must provide any particular medical treatment or health care benefit to its needy members. I shall suggest later that the level and type of provision can vary within certain reasonable boundaries according to the priorities determined by legitimate democratic procedures. The principle requires that if anyone within a society has an opportunity to receive a service or good that satisfies a health need, then everyone who shares the same type and degree of health need must be given an equally effective chance of receiving that service or good.

Since this is a principle of equal *access*, it does not guarantee equal *results*, although it would probably move our society in that direction. Discriminations in health care are permitted if they are based upon type or degree of health need, willingness of informed adults to be treated, and choices of life-style among the population. The equal-access principle constrains the distribution of opportunities to receive health care to an egalitarian standard, but it does not determine the total level of health care available or the effects of that care (provided the care is of equal quality) upon the health of the population. Of course, even if equality in health care were defined according to an "equal health" principle,[2] one would still have to admit—given the unequal distribution of illness among people and our present medical knowledge—that a just health care system could not come close to producing an equally healthy population.

Practical Implications

Since the equal-access principle requires equality of effective opportunity to receive care, not merely equality of formal legal

[2]Robert M. Veatch, "What Is a 'Just' Health Care Delivery?" in *Ethics and Health Policy*, ed. by Robert M. Veatch and Roy Branson (Cambridge, Mass.: Ballinger, 1976), pp. 127–53.

access, it does not permit discriminations based upon those characteristics of people that we can reasonably assume they did not freely choose. Such characteristics include sex, race, genetic endowment, wealth, and, often, place of residence. Even in an ideal society, equally needy persons will not use the same amount or quality of health care. Their preferences and their knowledge will differ, as will the skills of the providers who treat them.

A One-Class System

The most striking result of applying the equal-access principle in the United States would be the creation of a one-class system of health care. Services and goods that meet health care needs would be equally available to everyone who was equally needy. As a disincentive to overuse, only small fees for service could be charged for health care—provided that charges did not prove a barrier to entry to the poorest people who were needy. A one-class system need not, of course, be a uniform system. Diversity among medical and health care services would be permissible, indeed even desirable,[3] as long as the diversity did not create differential access along nonconsensual lines such as wealth, race, sex, or geographical location.

Equal access also places limits upon the market freedoms of some individuals, especially, but not exclusively, the richest members of society. The principle does not permit the purchase of health care to which other similarly needy people do not have effective access. The extent to which freedom of the rich must be restricted will depend upon the level of public provision for health care and the degree of income inequality. As the level of health care guaranteed to the poor decreases and the degree of

[3]Paul Starr, "A National Health Program: Organizing Diversity," *The Hastings Center Report*, V (1975), 11–13.

income inequality increases, the equal-access standard demands greater restrictions upon the market freedom of the rich. Where income and wealth are very unevenly distributed and where the level of access publicly guaranteed is very low, the rich can use the market to buy access to health care goods unavailable to the poor, thereby undermining the effective equality of opportunity required by an equal-access principle.

The restriction on market freedoms to purchase health care under these circumstances creates a certain discomforting irony: the equal-access principle permits—or is at least agnostic with respect to—the free-market satisfaction of preferences for nonessential consumer goods. Thus, the rigorous implementation of equal access to health care would restrict rich people from spending their extra income for preferred medical services if those services were not equally accessible to the poor. It would not restrict them from using those same resources to purchase satisfactions in other areas—a Porsche or any other luxurious consumer goods. In discussing additional problems created by an attempt to implement a principle of equal access to health care in an otherwise inegalitarian society, I return later to consider whether advocates of equal access can avoid this irony.

Hard Cases

As with all principles, hard cases exist for the equal-access principle. Without dwelling upon these cases, it is worth considering how the principle might deal with two hard but fairly common cases: therapeutic experimentation in medicine and alternative treatments of different quality.

Each year in the United States, many potentially successful therapies are tested. Since their value has not been proved, there may be good reason to limit their use to an appropriate sample of sick experimental subjects. The equal-access principle would insist that experimenters choose these subjects at random from a population of relevantly sick consenting adults. A randomized clinical trial could be advertised by public notice, and individuals who were interested might be registered and enrolled on a lottery basis. The only requirement for enrollment would be the health conditions and personal characteristics necessary for proper scientific testing.

How does one apply the principle of equal access when alternative treatments are each functionally adequate but aesthetically or socially quite disparate? Take the hypothetical case of a societal commitment to adequate dentition among adults. Replacement of carious or mobile teeth with dentures may preserve dental function at relatively minor cost. On the other hand, full mouth reconstruction, involving periodontal and endodontal treatment and capping of affected teeth, may be only marginally more effective but substantially more satisfying. The added costs for the preferred treatment are not inconsiderable. The principle would seem to demand that at equal states of dental need there by equal access to the preferred treatment. However, it is unclear whether the satisfaction of subjective desire is equivalent to fulfillment of objective need.

In cases of alternative treatments, proponents of equal access could turn to another argument for providing access to the same treatments for all. A society that publicly provides the minimal acceptable treatment freely to all and also permits a private market in more expensive treatments may result in having a two-class system of care. The best providers will service the richest clientele, thereby risking less-than-adequate treatment for the poorest. Approval of a private market in alternative treatments would rest upon the empirical hypothesis that if the publicly funded level of adequate treatment were high enough, few people would choose to short circuit the public (i.e., equal access) sector; the small additional free-market sector would not threaten to lower the quality of services that were universally available. Most cases, like the one of dentistry, are difficult to decide merely on principle. Proponents of equal access must take into account the consequences of alternative policies. But empirical knowledge alone will not decide these issues, and arguments for or against a particular policy can be entertained in a more systematic way once one exposes the values that underlie support for an equal-access principle. One can then judge to what extent alternative policies satisfy these values.

Supporting Values

Advocates of equal access to health care must demonstrate why health care is different from other consumer goods, unless they are willing to support the more radical principle of equal distribution of all goods. Norman Daniels[4] provides one foundation for distinguishing between health care and other goods. He establishes a category of health care needs whose satisfaction provides an important condition for future opportunity. Like police protection and education, some kinds of health care goods are necessary for pursuing most other goods in life. Any theory of justice committed to equalizing opportunity ought to treat health care as a good deserving of special distributive treatment. Equal access to health care provides a necessary, although certainly not a sufficient, condition for equal opportunity in general.

A precept of egalitarian justice that physical pains of a sufficient degree be treated similarly regardless of who experiences them establishes another reason for singling out certain kinds of

[4]Norman Daniels, "Health-Care Needs and Distributive Justice," *Philosophy and Public Affairs*, X (1981), 146–79.

health care as speical goods.[5] Some health conditions cause great
pain but are not linked to a serious curtailment of opportunity.
The two values are, however, mutually compatible.

A theory of justice that gives priority to the value of equal
respect among people might also be used to support a principle
of equal access to health care. John Rawls, for example, argues
that without self-respect "nothing may seem worth doing, or if
some things have value for us, we lack the will to strive for them.
. . .Therefore the parties in the original position would wish to
avoid at almost any cost the social conditions that undermine self-
respect."[6]

Conditions of Self-respect

It is not easy to determine what social conditions support or
undermine self-respect. One might plausibly assume that equalizing opportunity and treating similar pains similarly would be
the most essential supports for equal respect within a health care
system. And so, in most cases, the value of equal respect provides
additional support for equal access to the same health care goods
that are warranted by the values of equal opportunity and relief
from pain. But at least some kinds of health care treatment not
essential to equalizing opportunity or bringing equal relief from
pain may be necessary to equalize respect within a society. It is
conceivable that much longer waiting time in physicians' offices
or for admission to hospitals may not affect the long-term health
prospects of the poor or blacks. But such discriminations in waiting times for an essential good probably do adversely affect the
self-respect of those who systematically stand at the end of the
queue.

[5]For the theoretical foundations of such a precept, see Amy Gutmann, *Liberal
Equality* (New York: Cambridge University Press, 1980), pp. 20–27.
[6]*A Theory of Justice* (Cambridge, Mass.: Harvard University Press, 1971), p. 440.

Some of the conditions necessary for equal respect are socially relative; we must arrive at a standard of equal respect appropriate to our particular society. Universal suffrage has long been a condition for equal respect; the case for it is independent of the anticipated results of equalizing political power by granting every person one vote. More recently, equal access to health care has similarly become a condition for equal respect in our society. Most of us do not base our self-respect on the way we are treated on airplanes, even though the flight attendants regularly give preferential treatment to those traveling first class. This contrast with suffrage and health care treatment (and education and police protection) no doubt is related to the fact that these goods are much more essential to our security and opportunities in life than is airplane travel. But it is still worth considering that unequal treatment in health care, as in education, may be understood as a sign of unequal respect even where there are no discernible adverse effects on the health or education of those receiving less favored treatment. Even where a dual health care system will not produce inferior medical results for the less privileged, the value of equal respect militates against the perpetuation of such a system in our society.

Challenges

Equality of opportunity, equal relief from pain, and equal respect are the three central values providing the foundation of support for a principle of equal access to health care. Any theory of justice that gives primacy to these values (as do many liberal and egalitarian theories) will lend prima facie support to a health care system structured along equal-access lines.

We are now in a position to consider alternative values and empirical claims that would lead someone to challenge, or reject, a principle of equal access to health care. These challenges also enable us to elaborate further the moral and political implications of the principle.

Proponents of the Market

The most radical and vocal opposition comes from those who support a pure free-market principle in health care. A foundation of support for the free-market principle is the idea that the relative importance of satisfying different human desires is a purely subjective matter: we can distinguish between one person's desire for good medical care and another person's desire for a good Beaujolais only by the price they are willing to pay for each. If no goods are special because there is no way of ranking desires except by individual processes of choice, then what better way than the unconstrained market to allow us to decide among the smorgasbord of goods society has to offer?[7]

Health care goods and services are likely to be more equally allocated through the market if income and wealth are more equally distributed. Several defenders of the market as a means of allocating goods and services also support a moderate degree of income redistribution on grounds of its diminishing marginal utility or because they believe that every person has a right to a "basic minimum."[8] Neither rationale for redistribution takes us very far toward a principle of equal access to health care. If one retains the basic assumption that human preferences are totally

[7]See Charles Fried, "Health Care, Cost Containment, Liberty" (paper presented to the Institute of Society, Ethics and the Life Sciences, Hastings-on-Hudson, New York, 1979); Robert Nozick, *Anarchy, State and Utopia* (New York: Basic Books, 1974); and Robert M. Sade, "Medical Care as a Right: A Refutation," *New England Journal of Medicine*, CCLXXXV (1971), 1288–92.

[8]See Milton Friedman, *Capitalism and Freedom* (Chicago: Chicago University Press, 1962); and Charles Fried, *Right and Wrong* (Cambridge, Mass.: Harvard University Press, 1978).

subjective, then the market remains the best way to order human priorities. Only the market appropriately decentralizes decision making and eliminates all nonconsensual exchanges of goods and services.[9]

Although a minimum income floor under all individuals increases *access* to most goods and services, even at a higher level than that supported by Friedman and others, a guaranteed income will be inadequate to sustain the costs of a catastrophic illness. A *very* high guaranteed minimum might result in almost universal insurance coverage at a fairly high level. Supporters of free-market allocation do not, however, press for a very high minimum for at least two reasons. They fear its effects on incentives and they cannot justify a high guaranteed income without admitting that there are many expensive goods that are not just mere consumer preferences but essential to all persons.

The first reason for opposing a very high minimum is probably a good one. A principle approaching equality of income and wealth is likely to have serious disincentive effects on productive work and investment. There are also better reasons for treating health care as a special good—a good that society has an obligation to provide equally to all its members—than there are for distributing most consumer goods equally.

A significant step beyond the pure free-market principle is a position that preserves the role of the market in allocating different "packages" of health care according to consumer preferences but concedes a role for government in supplying every adult with a "voucher" of a certain monetary value redeemable exclusively for health care goods and services. Proponents of health vouchers must assume that there is something special about health care to justify government in taxing its citizens to provide universally for these goods and not all others. But if health

[9]Fried, *Right and Wrong*, pp. 124–26.

care is a more important good, because it preserves life and
expands opportunity, then what is the rationale for effectively
limiting the demand a sick but poor person can make upon the
health care system? Why should access to health care be dependent upon income or wealth at all?

Opponents of equal access generally imply that more than
minimal access will unjustly curtail the freedom of citizens as
taxpayers, as consumers, and as providers of health care. Let us
consider seperately the arguments with regard to the many citizens who are taxpayers and consumers and the few who are
providers of health care.

The Charge of Paternalism

Charles Fried has argued that equal access to health care is
a particularly intrusive form of paternalism toward citizens. Fried
claims further that "apart from a rather general commitment to
equality and, indeed, to state control of the allocation and distribution of resources, to insist on the right to health care, where
that right means a right to equal access, is an anomaly. For as
long as our society considers that inequalities of wealth and income are morally acceptable . . .it is anomalous to carve out a
sector like health care and say that *there* equality must reigh."[10]

Would an equal access system necessarily be intrusive or
paternalistic in its operation? A national health care system simply
cannot be said to take away the income entitlement of citizens,
since citizens are not entitled to their gross incomes. We can
determine our income entitlement only after we deduct from our
gross income the amount we owe the state to support the rights
of others. To the extent that the rationale of an equal-access

[10]Fried, "Equality and Rights in Medical Care," *Hastings Center Report*, VI
    (1976), 31.

principle is redistributive, those individuals who otherwise could not afford certain health care services will experience an expansion of their freedom (assuming an adequate level of social provision). Of course, part of the justification of a national health care system is that it would also guarantee health care coverage to people who could afford adequate health care but who would not be prudent enough to save or to invest in insurance. Even if we accept the common definition of paternalistic actions as those that restrict an individual's liberty so as to further his or her interest, we still have to assess the assertion that this (partial) rationale for an equal-access system entails a restriction of individual liberty. Unlike a law banning the sale of cigarettes or forcing people to wear seat belts, the institution of a national health care system forces no one to use it. If a majority of citizens decide that they want to be taxed in order to ensure themselves health care, the resulting legislation could not be considered paternalistic:

> Legislation requiring contributions to some cooperative scheme (such as medical care). . .is not necessarily paternalistic, so long as its purpose is to give effect to the desires of a democratic majority, rather than simply to coerce a minority who do not want the benefits of the legislation.[11]

It is significant in this regard that, for the past 20 years, the Michigan Survey of registered voters has found a consistent and solid majority supporting government measures designed to ensure universal access to medical care.

The charge of paternalism levied against an equal-access system is therefore dubious because it is extremely difficult, if not impossible, to isolate the self-protectionist rationale from the redistributive and the democratic rationales. Those who object to a national health care system on the grounds that it is coercing

[11]Dennis F. Thompson, "Paternalism in Medicine, Law and Public Policy," *Ethics Teaching in Higher Education*, ed. by Daniel Callahan and Sissela Bok (New York: Plenum Press, 1980), p. 247.

some people for their own good forget that such a system still could be justified as a means to avoid the threat to a one-class system that exempting the rich would create. To condemn such a system as paternalistic would commit us to criticizing all legislation in which a democratic majority decides to protect itself against the wishes of a minority whose exemption from the resulting policy would undermine it. Other critics wrongly assume that people have an entitlement to the cash equivalent of the medical care to which society grants them a right. People do not have such an entitlement because taxpayers have a right to demand that their tax dollars be spent to satisfy health needs, not to buy luxuries. Indeed, our duty to pay taxes is dependent upon the fact that certain needs of other people must be given priority over our own desires for a more commodious style of life.

Other Restrictions

Nonetheless, two restrictions on consumer freedom are entailed in an equal-access system. One is the restriction imposed by the taxation necessary to provide all citizens, but especially the poorest, with access to health care goods. This restriction does not raise unique or particularly troublesome moral problems as long as one believes that the freedom to retain one's gross income is not an absolute right and that the resulting redistribution of income to the health care sector increases the life chances and thereby the effective freedom of many citizens.

But there is a second restriction of consumer market freedom sanctioned by the equal access principle: the limitation on freedom to buy health care goods above the level publicly provided. Aside from reasserting the primary values of equality, there is at least one plausible argument for such a restriction. Without restricting the free market in extra health care goods, a society risks having its best medical practitioners drained into the private market sector, thereby decreasing the quality of medical care received by the majority of citizens confined to the publicly funded sector. The lower the level of public provision of health care and the less elastic the supply of physicians, the more problematic from the perspective of the values underlying equal access will be an additional market sector in health care.

Without an additional market sector, would the freedom of physicians and other providers to practice wherever and for whomever they choose be unduly restricted? The extent of such restrictions will also vary with the level of public provision and with the diversity of the health care system. Public funds are already crucial to providing many physicians with basic income (through Medicare and Medicaid fees), research opportunities (through NIH), and hospitals and other institutions in which to practice (through Hill–Burton). In place of the time and resources now directed to privately purchased add-ons, an equal access system would redirect providers toward meeting previously unserved needs. These types of redirections of supply and redistributions of demand are commonly accepted in other professions that are oriented toward satisfying an important public interest. The legal and teaching professions are analogous in this regard. The equal-access principle, strictly interpreted, however, adds another restriction, a limitation upon private practice that supplies health care goods not equally accessible to the entire population of relevantly needy persons. This restriction upon the freedom of providers does not have an analogue in the present practice of law or of education, although the arguments for equal access to the goods of these professions might be similar. Therefore one's assessment of the strength of the case for such a restriction is likely to have implications beyond the health care system.

It is hard to see why one ought to prevent people, rich or poor, from spending money on health care goods while permitting them to spend money on consumer goods that are clearly not essential and perhaps even detrimental to health. One reason might be the possible systemic effect, mentioned above, of such additional expenditures in depriving the less advantaged of the best physicians. The freedom of providers as well as consumers would have to be restricted in order to curtail this effect. But beyond this empirically contingent argument for restricting any market in health care goods that are not equally accessible to all, the strict limitations upon market freedom in "extra" health care goods are hard to accept if one believes that medical services are at least as worthy items of expense as other consumer goods. One could argue that physicians ought to be free to meet the demand for additional medical goods, especially when that demand is a substitute for demand for less important goods.

This criticism illuminates a more general problem of attempting to equalize access to any good in an otherwise inegalitarian society. The more unequal the distribution of income and wealth within our society, the more likely it is that the freedom of consumers and providers to buy and sell health care outside the publicly funded sector will result in inequalities that cannot properly be regarded merely as the product of differences in consumer preferences. Therefore, in an inegalitarian society, we must live with a moral tension between granting providers the freedom to leave the publicly funded sector and achieving more equality in the satisfaction of health care needs.

A principle of equal access to health care applied within an otherwise egalitarian society might give little or no reason to restrict the freedom of providers or consumers. One argument often voiced against a publicly funded system that permits a marginal free-market sector is that the government is a less efficient provider of goods than are private parties. But the equal-access principle does not require that the government directly provide medical services through, for example, a national health service. Government need only be a regulator of the use and distribution of essential health care goods and services. This is a role that most people concede to government for many other purposes deemed essential to the welfare of all individuals.

Government regulation may, of course, be more expensive and hence less efficient than government provision of health care services of similar extent and quality. The tradeoff here would be between the additional market choice facilitated by government regulation of private providers and the decreased public cost of government provision. Despite utilitarian claims to the contrary, no simple moral calculus exists that would enable an impartial spectator to determine where the balance of advantage lies. Philosophers ought to cede to a fairly constituted democratic majority the right to decide this issue. What constitutes a fair process of democratic decision making is an important question of procedural justice that lies beyond this paper.

Liability for Voluntary Risks?

Another important criticism of the equal access principle cuts across advocacy of the free market and of government regulation of health care. Supporters of both might consistently ask whether it is fair to provide the same level of access for all people, including those who voluntarily adopt bad health habits and who quite knowingly and willingly take greater than average risks with their lives and health. Even if it might be unjust not to provide health care for those people once the need arises, why would it not be fair to force those who choose to drink, smoke, rock climb, and skydive also to bear a greater burden of their ensuing medical costs than that borne by people who deliberately avoid these risky pursuits? An equal-access principle seems to neglect the distinction between voluntary and nonvoluntary health risks in its eagerness to ensure that all people have an equal opportunity to receive appropriate health care.

Gerald Dworkin extensively and convincingly argues that it would not be unfair to force individuals to be financially liable for voluntarily undertaken health risks, but only under certain conditional assumptions. [12] These include our ability (1) to determine the relative causal role of voluntary versus nonvoluntary factors in the genesis of illness, (2) to differentiate between purely voluntary behavior and that which is nonvoluntary or compulsive, and (3) to distinguish between genetic and nongenetic predispositions to illness. For example, to satisfy the first condition, one would have to determine the relative causal role of smoking and environmental pollution in the genesis of cancer; to fulfill the second, one must know when smoking (or drinking or obesity) is voluntary and when it is compulsive behavior; and to satisfy the third condition, one must distinguish among those who smoke and get cancer and those who smoke and do not. In addition, as long as there are no good institutional mechanisms for monitoring certain risky activities or for differentiating between moderate and immoderate users of unhealthy substances, qualifying the equal-access principle to take account of voluntary health risks is likely to create more unfairness rather than less. Finally, given great inequalities in income distribution, the poor will be less able to bear the consequences of their risky behavior than will the rich, creating a situation of unfairness at least as serious as the unfairness of equally distributing the burdens of health care costs between those who voluntarily impose risks on themselves and those who do not. With respect to the health hazards of overeating and obesity, for example, the rich have recourse to expensive programs of weight control unavailable to the poor.

[12]"Responsibility and Health Risks," (paper presented to the Institute of Society, Ethics and the Life Sciences, Hastings-on-Hudson, New York, 1979).

Since we have such scanty knowledge of situations when sickness can be attributed to voluntary health risks, criticisms of the equal-access principle from this perspective have more weight in principle than they do in practice.

Equal Access to All Health Goods

All criticisms considered so far are directed at the equal-access principle from a perspective suggesting that government involvement and public funding of health care would be too great and the role of the market too small in an equal access system. Now let us consider a powerful criticism of the principle for including too little, rather than too much, in the public sector. The criticism can be posed in the form of a challenge: if one crucial reason for supporting a principle of equal access is that health goods are much more essential than many other goods because they provide a basis for equalizing opportunity and relieving substantial pain, then why not require a government to provide equal access to *all* those health goods that would move a society further in the direction of equalizing opportunity and relieving pain for the physically and mentally ill? Without pretending that our society could ever arrive at a condition of absolute equality of health (or therefore strict equality of opportunity), proponents of this principle could still argue that we should move as far as possible in that direction.

In a society in which no tradeoffs had to be made between health care and other goods, equal access to *all* health goods might be the most acceptable principle of equity in health care.[13] Of course, we do not live in such a society. Given the advanced state of our medical and health care technology and the prevalence of acute degenerative diseases and mental disorders in our population, a requirement that society provide access to every

---

[13]Veatch, "What is a 'Just' Health Care Delivery?" pp. 127–53.

known health care good would place an enormous drain upon
social resources.[14]

Costliness *per se* is not the main issue. The problem with
the principle of equal access to all health goods is that it demands
an absolute tradeoff between satisfaction of health care needs and
other needs and desires. The simplest argument against this principle is that other needs—such as education, police protection,
and legal aid—will be sacrificed to health care if the principle is
enforced. But this argument is too simple. A proponent of equal
access to all health goods could consistently establish some priority among these goods, all of which satisfy needs derived in large
part from a principle of equal opportunity. The weightier coun-
terargument is that above some less than maximum level in the
provision of opportunity goods, it seems reasonable for people
to value what, for want of a better term, one might call "quality
of life" goods: cultural, recreational, noninstrumental educational
goods and even consumer amenities. A society that maximized
the satisfaction of needs before it even began to provide access
to "quality of life" goods would be a dismal society indeed. Most
people do not want to devote their entire lives to being maximally
secure and healthy. Why, then, should a society devote all of its
resources to satisfying human *needs*?

Democracy and Equal Access

We need to find some principle or procedure by which to
draw a line at an appropriate level of access to health care short
of what is socially and technologically possible but greater than
what an unconstrained market would afford to most people, particularly to the least advantaged. I suspect that no philosophical

---

[14]For an account of changing patterns in health care in the United States, see
Anne R. Somers, *Health Care in Transition: Directions for the Future* (Chicago:
Hospital Research and Educational Trust, 1971), chap. 2.

argument can provide us with a cogent principle by which we can draw a line within the enormous group of goods that can improve health or extend the life prospects of individuals.

This problem of determining a proper level of guaranteed social satisfaction of need is not unique to health care. Something similar can be said about police protection or education in our society. Philosophers can provide reasons why police protection and education are rightly considered basic collective needs and why they should be given priority over individual consumer preferences. But no plausible philosophical principle can tell us what level of police protection or how much education a society ought to provide on an egalitarian basis.

The principle of equal access to health care establishes a criterion of distribution for whatever level of health care a society provides for any of its members. And further philosophical argument might establish some criteria by which to judge when the publicly funded level of health care was so low as to be unfair to the least advantaged or so high as to create undue restrictions on the ability of most people to live interesting and fulfilling lives. The remaining question of establishing a precise level of priorities among health care and other goods (at the "margin") is appropriately left to democratic decision making. The advantage of the democratic process in determining the precise level of health care provision is that citizens have an equal and collective voice in determining a decision that, according to the equal-access principle, ought to be mutually binding. Citizens not only reap the benefits but also share the burdens of the decision to expand or limit access to health care.

There is yet another advantage to this procedural method of establishing a fair level of health care provision. If the democratic decision will be binding on all citizens, as the equal-access principle assumes it must be, then one might expect the most advantaged citizens to exercise more political pressure to increase access to health care and hence increase the opportunity of the least advantaged above the level that they could afford in a free-market system or in a system where the rich were not included within the publicly funded health care sector. One finds some evidence to support this hypothesis in comparing the relative immunity from budget cutbacks of the program under universal entitlement of Medicare compared to the income-related Medicaid program. Of course, if costliness to the taxpayer is one's only concern, this added political pressure for health care expenditures is a liability rather than a strength of a one-class system. But from the perspective of equal access, the cost of a two-class system, one privately and one publicly funded, is an inequitable distribution of quantity and quality of care according to wealth, not need. The added nonproductive costs required merely to keep the two classes apart are seldom taken into account. And from the perspective of those supporters of an equal-access principle who also want to increase the total level of health care provision, the two-class system threatens to work in the opposite direction, siphoning off the pressure of citizens who have a disproportionate share of political influence. A democratic decision, the results of which are constrained by the principle of equal access, will give a relatively accurate reading of what most people believe to be an adequate level of health care protection. The major disadvantage of the equal-access constraint is that the decision of the majority or its representatives binds everyone, even those people who want more than the socially mandated level of health care.

Given the great economic inequalities of our society, it is politically impossible for advocates of equal access to fulfill their task. No democratic legislator could possibly succeed in winning support for a proposal that restricted market freedom as extensively as a strict interpretation of the equal-access principle requires. And it probably would be a mistake to insist upon strict philosophical standards: one thereby risks throwing the possibility of greater access to health care for the poor out with the insistence upon curtailing access for the rich.

Conclusion

I began by arguing that a principle of equal access to health care was at best an ideal toward which our society might strive. I shall end by qualifying that statement. A sufficiently high level of public provision of health care for all citizens and a sufficiently elastic supply of health care would significantly reduce the threat to universal provision of quality health care of a private market in extra health care goods, just as a very high level of police protection and education reduces the inequalities of opportunity resulting from purchase of private bodyguards or of prep school education by the rich.

In the best of all imaginable worlds of egalitarian justice, the equal-access principle would be sufficiently supported by other egalitarian economic and political institutions that a market in health care would complement rather than undercut the goals of equal respect and opportunity. In our society, the best that we can reasonably hope to achieve is a more universal and higher level of health care coupled with a greater supply of qualified primary care physicians and paramedics. These measures alone will not satisfy the equal-access principle, but they would move us a long way toward fulfilling those ideals that inform support for equal access. It is politically infeasible as well as morally problematic to fulfil the equal-access principle by restricting the market in health care goods above the guaranteed social minimum. Recognition of the limits of partial distributive justice thus requires that we be prepared to live with moral deficiencies within a system of health care as long as we live within a fundamentally inegalitarian society. Given the effects of economic and political inequalities upon the distribution of health care in the United States, our best alternative is to strive for imperfection.

ACKNOWLEDGMENTS

I am grateful to the members of the Hastings Center Group and especially to Norman Daniels, Gerald Dworkin, David Willis, and Daniel Wikler for helpful suggestions.

References

Daniels, N. "Equity of Access to Health Care: Some Conceptual and Ethical Issues." Paper presented to The President's Commission for the Study of Ethical Issues in Medicine and Biomedical and Behavioral Research, Washington, D.C., 1981.

Daniels, N. "Health-Care Needs and Distributive Justice." *Philosophy and Public Affairs*, X (1981);146–79.

Dworkin, Gerald. "Responsibility and Health Risks." Paper presented to the Institute of Society, Ethics and the Life Sciences, Hastings-on-Hudson, New York, 1979.

Fried, C. "Equality and Rights in Medical Care." *Hastings Center Report*, VI (1976);30–32.

Fried, C. "Difficulties in the Economic Analysis of Rights." *Markets and Morals*. Edited by G. Dworkin, G. Bermant, and P. G. Brown. Washington, D.C.: Hemisphere Publishing, 1977; pp. 175–95.

Fried, C. *Right and Wrong*. Cambridge, Mass.: Harvard University Press, 1978.

Fried, C. "Health Care, Cost Containment, Liberty." Paper presented to the Institute of Society, Ethics and the Life Sciences, Hastings-on-Hudson, New York, 1979.

Friedman, M. *Capitalism and Freedom*. Chicago: University of Chicago Press, 1962.

Gutmann, A. *Liberal Equality*. New York: Cambridge University Press, 1980.

Nozick, R. *Anarchy, State and Utopia*. New York: Basic Books, 1974.

Rawls, J. *A Theory of Justice*. Cambridge, Mass.: Harvard University Press, 1971.

Sade, Robert N. "Medical Care as a Right: A Refutation." *New England Journal of Medicine*, CCLXXXV (1971), 1288–92.

Somers, Anne R. *Health Care in Transition: Directions for the Future*. Chicago: Hospital Research and Educational Trust, 1971.

Starr, P. "A National Health Program: Organizing Diversity." *The Hastings Center Report,* V (1975); 11–13.

Thompson, Dennis F. "Paternalism in Medicine, Law and Public Policy." *Ethics Teaching in Higher Education.* Edited by D. Callahan and S. Bok. New York: Plenum Press, 1980.

Veatch, Robert M. "What Is a 'Just' Health Care Delivery?" *Ethics and Health Policy.* Edited by R. M. Veatch and Roy Branson. Cambridge, Mass.: Ballinger, 1976, pp. 127–53.

3

Nancy Neveloff Dubler

Jail and Prison Health Care Standards

A DETERMINATION OF NEED WITHOUT REFERENCE
TO WANT OR DESIRE

Introduction

Delivering health care in a jail or prison is delivering care in a
"non-health-care space." Health care professionals must diagnose, treat, care for, and comfort in an institution designed to
confine, humiliate, infantilize, punish, and reform. The intrinsic
conflict between the goals of a health care delivery system and
the goals of penal institutions has historically produced and continues now to create most severe tensions in the interactions
between correctional personnel and health care providers and it
also challenges the relationship usually assumed to exist between
providers and their patients.

The disharmony between the goals of health care and the
tasks of prisons—that is, between the medical model and the
penal model—has come into bright relief since the growth and
development of the concept of the penitentiary in the 1700s,

Nancy Neveloff Dubler ● Department of Social Medicine, Montefiore Medical
Center, Bronx, New York 10467.

although there were anticipations in the preceding centuries. Pre-eighteenth-century imprisonment, however, was an infrequent punishment used for those in great disfavor, disrepute, or political disgrace for whom execution was impractical. Those imprisoned, it was assumed, would most probably perish in their castle dungeon or tower cell; Daniel, when placed in the lion's den, had little expectation of humane care and treatment.

Thus, until quite recently, imprisonment was most often designed to inflict suffering and death; no one expected—indeed it would have been ludicrous to suggest, let alone demand—that among the jailer's obligations was the preservation and support of the health and well-being of the jailed. Torture, often sanctioned by both state and church, was in many societies the accepted and approved way of dealing with the jailed; the object of prison was not to confine without "cruel and unusual" punishment but, on the contrary, to create a setting in which the viciousness of the human spirit could find free and lawful expressions.

In England, the late eighteenth century saw not only social, political, and economic realignments but also a new kind of enlightenment and reformist philosophy, all of which led to the increased use of imprisonment in the new form of the penitentiary.[1] At the same time in America, the framers of the Constitution rejected torture, long associated with the excessess of the monarchy, and prohibited "cruel and unusual" punishments. In addition, and very practically, America closed its doors to minor criminals sentenced to "transportation" from England, thus necessitating some increased ability to "punish" in England itself.

Early-eighteenth-century punishment had relied heavily on public ritual and called for harsh deterrents—including use of

---

[1]For a general discussion of the growth and development of the modern penitentiary, see Michael Ignatieff, *A Just Measure of Pain: The Penitentiary in the Industrial Revolution, 1750–1850* (New York: Pantheon Books, 1978).

the pillory, whipping, and executions—that were often mitigated in particular cases by judicial decree. As crime began to increase and become more visible, new theories of deterrence and reform gained acceptance and the modern penitentiary took form. These prisons were based on a theoretical commitment to moral reformation which rendered inappropriate ancient methods of physical torture. A society using dungeons designed for torture can accept prisoner deaths as a justifiable "cost of doing business"; however, a setting for reform must keep penitents alive and well as a precondition to success. Thus the penitentiary needed *some* modicum of health care to fulfill its goals, but it was an uneasy alliance from the beginning. The development of standards for prison health and the controversy over their appropriateness for care is merely the latest manifestation of the struggle to mate an elephant and a goose in the hopes of producing a viable offspring.

The struggle to introduce regular medical supervision into the English penitentiaries in the 1780s describes the beginnings of modern prison health care. The Gloucestershire prisons were the most complete embodiment of the ideal of the penitentiary in the 1780s. They were committed to silence, separation, and moral reform. They were, in the main, the creation of one magistrate, Sir George Onefiphorous Paul. This magistrate, in his ongoing fashioning and supervision of the penitentiaries, became concerned with issues of hygiene mainly because of recurring epidemics of jail fever, which regularly decimated the prison population, and equally recurring epidemics of typhus, which were then exported to the surrounding community—with predictably disastrous results.

Magistrate Paul's difficulty, however, was his inability to convince fellow magistrates that the introduction of baths, uniforms, infirmaries for the sick, regular medical attention, better diet, and whitewashed walls would not compromise the pains of confinement. Paul's solution was to convince these magistrates that hygienic rituals could be made to serve punitive functions. Thus, for example, in a report to the justices in 1784, he suggested the shaving of convicts' heads, both as a measure of hygiene and as a salutary humiliation:

> I consider shaving the head as an important regulation first, because it infallibly cleanses the most filthy part of the person, and is the only means of preventing the introduction of vermin to the bedding. Secondly, because it changes the ordinary appearance of the person and goes far toward preventing prisoners from being recognized on their return to society, by those strangers who are daily admitted to a distant view of them when walking in the yards. And thirdly, because so far as shaving the head is a mortification to the offender, it becomes a punishment directed to the mind, and is (at least so I have conceived) an allowable alternative for inflicting corporal punishment intended to be excluded from the system.[2]

This articulation, which stood unopposed in the medical community, was the language of social and moral condemnation veiled as the language of medicine.[3] It was the beginning of the acceptance, by the medical profession, of the process by which ultimately the definitions of the responsibilities and the role of health professionals would be set by prison officials so as to fit in with the latter's goals.

This climate of moral condemnation was further supported by the social and class separation which, from its inception, characterized the modern penitentiary system. Physicians and magistrates were exclusively from the upper-middle and upper class; penitentiary inmates were almost entirely, in contrast to political prisoners of earlier centuries, the poor and unemployed. Their numbers increased, as now, in some relation to unemployment and social dislocation.

It is perhaps unfair to attack Sir George's initial justification

---

[2]Ibid., p. 100.
[3]Ibid., p. 60.

for the introduction of prison health services. For its time it was most probably the only acceptable or even conceivable justification for the introduction of medical care. The cost of introducing medical care was the subordination of the independent goals of the profession to the philosophy and needs of the prison or jail or penitentiary.

This "coopting" of medical care was relatively unimportant in the 1780s, when the benefits to inmates from the addition of any service, especially a health service, far outweighed any theoretical or practical objections to the relationship between that service and the prison administration. In recent years, however, it has become clear that this subservience may act to preclude the effective delivery of care.

The delivery of health care to inmates in underfunded, often physically inadequate, overcrowded, and understaffed institutions is a task that can only be accomplished by an independent and coequal health authority concerned exclusively with health needs of inmates. It is almost never convenient for correctional officials to vary schedules in order to provide access to routine care or to free staff for the extra security and transportation tasks necessary to obtain specialty care. Providing health care means constantly confronting the routine procedures, needs, budgets, and assumptions of prison administrators; this cannot be done effectively by a person subordinate to these administrators and therefore one concerned about his or her status, promotion, or continued employment. As in any labor–management situation, independence is the prerequisite for employee challenge. Over the decades, physicians and all medical staff came to be (where they even existed) regular employees of the prison. As such, they had neither the stature nor the courage to challenge prison regulations or rulings that were detrimental to their patients' general health or specific treatment plans.

Additionally, prison health workers and physicians did not

often have the stature, vision, and power of Sir George. The term "prison doc" has become in our society a term of derision and opprobrium. It implies an incompetent practitioner who is so bad he can work only with the filth of society and can deliver only the most inadequate of care. Unfortunately the term had often been a most accurate description. Whereas there are many reasons for the emergence of "prison docs," including inadequate renumeration, isolated and depressing facilities, and socially undesirable patients, a major barrier to the entrance of decent professionals into prison health care has been the knowledge that medical judgments and decisions (objectively determined medical needs) could be frustrated by nonmedical considerations. Because of this, medical determinations of need have had neither the objective basis nor the professional competence society has come to expect; a determination of patient need was colored by the reality of patient service.

The need for independent medical care has become more apparent as the oppressive nature and brutal operations of most prisons has become more clear. Thus modern prison medicine has concerned itself not with its prior history but with its present reform.

There are no clear statistics on how many men (women have always been few) were incarcerated in the English jails and prisons of the late eighteenth century. Today we have far more specific figures. The latest compiled statistics from the *National Prisoners Statistics Bulletin* show that there were 158,000 people held locally in the nation's jails in 1978, most either awaiting trial or serving short sentences of usually less than a year. They were disproportionately black (41%), male (94%), undereducated (three out of five had not completed high school), and under employed (43% were jobless prior to being jailed). The reported average income for this population demonstrated a median of $3,255 earned during the year prior to arrest.[4] In addition to those held in jails (mainly pretrial facilities), the most important population for the following discussion of jail standards, another approximately 200,000 individuals were incarcerated in 1978 in the nation's prisons (housing for sentenced individuals).

Penitentiaries were designed to be instruments for the segregation and moral reeducation of the unruly poor. In modern American society they may not serve precisely the same function, but they do serve precisely the same population. As such, they are institutions for the economically, socially, and medically most needy segment of our society.

The Modern Confrontation with Health Care in Prisons and Jails

Over the last decade there has been increasing discussion of the medical needs of incarcerated populations. A number of factors combined to focus attention on the deplorable lack of adequate medical care in prisons.

First, the civil rights and the antiwar movements created, for the first time since the Revolutionary War, a substantial number of middle-class, educated, and well-connected prisoners. Second, the Attica riot shocked the sensibility of a nation which, by inadvertence as much as by design, had placed prisons beyond the scope of outside scrutiny.

Most important, however, was the development of public-interest law firms and publicly funded attorneys, which permitted a small group of advocates in the early 1970s to bring court cases

[4]"Census of Jails and Survey of Jail Inmates, 1978," *National Prisoner Statistics Bulletin*, No. FD-NPS-J-6P (February), 1979.

that drew national attention to the abysmal level of medical care in many of the country's prisons and jails.

The paradigmatic case was *Newman* v. *Alabama*.[5] This was the first case to articulate the principle that practices within a prison system which result in the deprivation of basic elements of adequate medical treatment violate the Eighth Amendment's constitutional prohibition against cruel and unusual punishment; it further ruled that such practices could be examined, addressed, and prohibited by specifically drafted federal decree. *Newman* v. *Alabama* described a litany of horrors including medical care provided, supervised, and bartered by inmates; inmates left to die in their own filth; and surgery performed by uneducated and totally unprepared inmate health aides.

Newman v. *Alabama* occurred concurrent with the general demise of the "hands-off" doctrine, that exercise in judicial restraint which gave support, credence, and force of law to administrative discretion in the prisons; it had created another wall—one of silence and secrecy—which further surrounded the constraining wall of prisons. The hands-off doctrine, citing the intractibility of prison problems and their inappropriateness for judicial remediation, had given practically free rein to prison administrators.[6]

Therefore, one of the most significant aspects of the Newman decision was the specificity of the relief ordered. In addition to

[5]*Newman* v. *Alabama*, 349 F. Suppl. 278, 503 F. 2d, 1320 (5th Cir. 1974), Cert. denied 421 U.S. 948.

[6]For the abandonment of the hands-off doctrine, see *Procunier* v. *Martinez*, 416 U.S. 396, 404 (1973). "traditionally, federal courts have adopted a broad hands-off attitude toward problems of prison administration. . . . Suffice it to say that problems of prisons in America are complex and intractable and more to the point, they are not readily susceptible of resolution by decree . . . but a policy of judicial restraint cannot encompass any failure to take cognizance of valid constitutional claims whether arising in a federal or state institution. When a prison regulation or practice offends a fundamental constitutional guarantee, federal courts will discharge their duty to protect constitutional rights."

requiring penal administrators to submit their own plans for remedial action, the court ordered the general prison hospital in
Alabama to meet the standards that had been set by the federal
government for hospitals participating in and receiving funds from
Medicare. The court further ordered the hospital to comply with
the applicable regulations of the Federal Bureau of Narcotics and
Dangerous Drugs (FBNDD) and to hire a full-time medical director. Finally, it ordered that measures be taken to prevent
reprisals against inmates who had complained of illness, that
complete medical records for all inmates be organized and kept
separate from correctional records, and that an ambulance or
other vehicle be made available at all times to respond to medical
emergencies. Thus, in the earliest case dealing directly with modern medical care delivery systems in prison, the efforts of Federal
District Judge Frank M. Johnson were directed not only to the
relief of individual complaints but to the creation of *standards*
that could guide the future provision of health care service.

The cases following *Newman* v. *Alabama* continued to struggle with two separate kinds of definition. On the one hand, they
had to grapple with fact patterns that were intended to demonstrate "denial," "disregard," or "shockingly inadequate response"
(all phrases used in early cases) to the medical needs of inmates.
The words used to describe the incidents groped toward a legal
definition—legal standard—that could govern the deliberations
designed to determine whether there had been a constitutional
deprivation. Thus, the opinions held that there was "shocking,"
"abusive," "deliberately indifferent," or "inadequate" care. The
judgments or orders that followed these opinions struggled with
a different problem of definition, that of translating the developing constitutional standard—a retrospective legal rubric—into
operative standards or prospective practical guidelines. This was
obviously a most difficult and in some ways inappropriate task
for the federal judiciary.

78   NANCY NEVELOFF DUBLER

In grappling with the problems of creating a linguistic standard[7] able to reflect possible constitutional deprivations and a remedial standard able to ensure the proper provision of care, the federal courts had to fashion a standard broad enough to address the demonstrated evils in the system and yet narrow enough to avoid enmeshing the federal courts in an ongoing review of medical disputes (which is practically impossible) or the adjudication of allegations of malpractice (which is theoretically impossible, given the limits of federal jurisdiction). As this process unfolded, the medical establishment, prodded by congressional interest, became aware of and began to respond to the tales of horror emanating from the nation's prisons and jails.

While lawyers and judges were struggling to define the elements of a constitutional deprivation and the appropriate structure for remedial orders, government agencies (specifically the United States Department of Justice) and private organizations

[7]The linguistic war was finally won by the phrase "deliberate indifference," the language endorsed by the Supreme Court in Estelle v. Gamble, 429 U.S., 97, (1976), at 106:"Deliberate indifference to serious medical needs of prisoners constitutes the 'unnecessary and wanton infliction of pain' . . . proscribed by the Eighth Amendment. This is true whether the indifference is manifested by prison doctors in their response to the prisoner's needs or by prison guards in intentionally denying or delaying access to medical care or intentionally interfering with the treatment once proscribed. Regardless of how evidenced, deliberate indifference to a prisoner's serious illness or injury states a cause of action under section 1983 429 U.S. at 104–05. The deliberate indifference standard, however, was clarified by the Court to include only 'wanton infliction of unnecessary pain' and not an accident or inadverdent failure: Thus, a complaint that a physician has been negligent in diagnosing or treating a medical condition does not state a valid claim of medical mistreatment under the Eighth Amendment. Medical malpractice does not become a constitutional violation merely because the victim is a prisoner. In order to state a cognizable claim, a prisoner must allege acts or omissions sufficiently harmful to evidence deliberate indifference to serious medical needs. It is only such indifference that can offend 'evolving standards of decency' in violation of the Eighth Amendment" (429 U.S. at 106).

(preeminently the American Medical Association and the American Public Health Association) began to respond to the demonstrated need, spurred on by genuine concern, the personal interest of some highly placed individuals, and the offer of government funds to support research.

The 1970, the United States Department of Justice published a statistical survey of facilities in the nation's jails.[8] This survey first presented data on medical facilities in jails and demonstrated that well over half of the nation's jails had absolutely no provision for any kind of health care delivery for emergent, chronic, or acute conditions.

In response to this first brief and sketchy study, the American Medical Association conducted a more specific survey of 2,930 jails in mid-1972. The purpose of the survey was to determine "the medical resources and care available in United States jails as well as to assess the potential role of the medical profession in improving the care of inmate populations."[9]

This initial survey, conducted via questionnaires mailed to local sheriffs, produced 1,159 usable responses out of the almost 3,000 sent.[10] The results of the survey demonstrated again that most jails had woefully limited facilities for providing medical care to incarcerated populations: approximately 65% of the responding jails had only first aid facilities; 16.7% had no internal medical facilities, not even a first aid kit; in 50.6%, physicians were available on an on-call basis; and in 31.1%, no physicians were ever available to provide medical care to inmates. In almost

[8]U.S. Department of Justice, Law Enforcement Assistance Administration, National Criminal Justice Information and Statistics Service, *1970 National Jail Census* (Washington, D.C.: U.S. Government Printing Office, February, 1971).
[9]*Medical Care in U.S. Jails—A 1972 AMA Survey* (Chicago: AMA Division of Medical Practice, February, 1973), forward.
[10]Ibid.

all jails prescription drugs were dispensed to inmates who needed them (if they came with the medications), but in 81.6% of these the medications were dispensed by nonmedical personnel.[11]

These statistics, as the AMA clearly recognized, represented an enormous cost in human suffering. The survey proved definitively that there was a most immediate need for improvement of health care delivery in jails; the delivery capability was, in the majority of jails, nonexistent.

Based on the results of their survey, the Division of Medical Practice of the American Medical Association developed a document entitled *Proposal for a Program to Improve Medical Care and Health Services for Inmates of the Nation's Jails and Prisons and Juvenile Detention Facilities*.[12] The objects of the proposal were to stimulate an increased awareness of health care deficiencies in the nation's correctional institutions and to devise and undertake aggressive efforts to improve medical care within correctional systems. In support of these objectives, the proposal developed a schema of (1) evaluation, (2) establishment of guidelines and standards, and (3) use of those standards for the accreditation of individual programs. One problem stemmed from its initial assumption of a community of interest between prison health and correctional professionals, stating that "it's clear that officials within the corrections system share the desire of the AMA and the medical profession to improve health care and to achieve that goal in the shortest possible time."[13] Given the previous discussion on the need for medical independence, the AMA appears to have given insufficient weight to inevitable conflict. It assumed the cooperation of these professionals in the four phases

[11]Ibid., pp. ii and iii.
[12]Ibid.
[13]Ibid., p. 1.

of its program (i.e., compilation of data; communication of the need; coordination of medical, legal, and correctional improvement efforts; and certification of improved care).[14]

In June 1975, based on its proposal, the AMA received a grant from the Law Enforcement Assistance Administration to begin a program designed to improve the health care in the nation's jails. The development of jail health standards was one of the key goals of the initial stages of the program. During its first year of funding (which actually extended to the spring of 1977), the AMA worked with 30 pilot sites to develop model jail health delivery systems. The model sites were intended to test possible methods of improving care and to gather information on, and test the workability of, the developing standards.

Developing Standards for Correctional Health Care

As new models of service delivery were being tested, a national committee of experts from health and corrections was convened to develop a model set of standards for health care delivery in jails. (This group was largely made up of physicians, some nurses, and allied health professionals; it included no ex-offenders or inmate advocates.) Then began a three-year process during which standards were developed, tested in model sites, evaluated by these individual sites in conjunction with the standards committee, and finally retested in another site for appropriateness. The contractual evaluators of the project make the following interesting comment in their 1978 report: "Since the standards which were not met by a majority of the pilot sites could represent potential problems in accrediting jails in subsequent years, they

[14]Ibid., p. 4.

were isolated for review."[15] The report also stated that each procedural step in the accreditation process was examined for any
problems encountered by any of the sites in the original six states.

Again the profession appears to have been coopted. A health
care goal should not be accreditation but rather decent health
services; there is no necessary correlation between the two. However, the goal of correctional administrations, that of accreditation, invalidated certain of the more difficult-to-implement medical standards. This is not meant to imply that all or even most
prison administrators and correctional health providers are venal
or evil—merely that they are often understaffed, underfunded,
overwhelmed, and overburdened by society. They are expected
to cope without comment. The operation of the prisons in this
country may indeed provide new evidence of Hannah Arendt's
discussions of the "banality of evil."

By 1978, the AMA had isolated 42 items under which it
would assess the possibility of accreditation of local jails. Those
items were divided into the categories of "essential" and "important." In order for a jail to be accredited, it had to comply
fully with 90% of the essential requirements and with 80% of the
important standards. This, parenthetically, was a change from
the initial plan, under which a jail to be accredited would have
been required to comply with *all* the essential standards and 80%
of those remaining. However, in the process by which the standards were created, the reality of compliance tended to color the
necessity for change.

As Robert Brutsche, Medical Director for the Bureau of
Prisons (United States Public Health Service), stated the problem:

---

[15]B. Jaye Anno and Carlton A. Hornung, "Summary of an Evaluation of the
American Medical Association's *Program to Improve Health Care in Jails*" (paper
presented at the Second National Workshop on Criminal Justice Evaluation,
September, 1978), p. 6.

One of the prime problems in the early development of standards in any field is the dilemma of deciding whether the initial standards should be *minimal* with an *optimum* chance of attainment, or whether they should be *optimum* with a *minimum* chance of attainment. The latter approach results in standards which are unacceptable to the target organizations, except when compliance is not an option, i.e., when it is mandated by the courts. On the other hand, the development of *minimum* standards usually results in an incomplete set of guidelines which fails to accurately address the entire scope and depth of existing problems.[16]

Over the three years during which the standards were developed by the AMA, the responsible committee invited the participation of state medical society advisers, of special task forces, and of various members of the AMA national staff. In addition, they invited hundreds of sheriffs, jail administrators, and health care providers in jails across the country to comment on and contribute to the development of the standards. Thus, notes one commentator,

Despite the laudable and honest efforts of these groups, their standards and accreditation procedures must be recognized as the product of only one segment of those involved in prison health care—the providers.[17]

Thus, the development of prison health standards has reflected only the voice of professionals and professional societies:

Those most glaringly absent are the recipients of the care in custody—the inmates. The AMA did not really involve inmates or groups which represent them, nor has the AMA polled inmates to learn their priorities, their ideas of how to improve care, or their views on what mechanisms for monitoring are needed.[18]

[16]Robert L. Brutsche, "Medical Standards for Corrections: A Status Report." *Corrections Today*, July–August, 1979.

[17]Judith Resnik and Nancy Shaw, "Prisoners of Their Sex, Health Problems of Incarcerated Women," *A Prisoner's Rights Source Book: Theory, Litigation and Practice*, Vol. II. edited by Ira Robbins (New York: Clark Boardman, Inc. 1980), p. 77.

[18]Ibid., p. 76.

This paper has examined the process by which the AMA standards were developed at some length, notwithstanding the fact that they were developed subsequent to earlier sets of standards which were published by the American Public Health Association (APHA) and the Law Enforcement Assistance Administration.[19] These earlier sets of standards received little support although they were interesting and, indeed, in the case of the APHA standards, much broader in their definition of public health needs of inmates and the probable risk factors associated with the process of incarceration itself (e.g., overcrowding and inadequate sanitation). Whereas the APHA standards have at times been used by various federal judges seeking to fashion specific decrees or to provide ongoing guidance to federal "masters," the simpler and less challenging AMA standards (with their accompanying promise of accreditation) have been far more widely used and recognized both by practitioner groups and by the courts. Thus, despite noted process deficiencies, the AMA, linking standards with accreditation, established an incentive for jails first to evaluate and then to confront the inadequacies of their system, thus beginning to bring change.

Analysis of Standards

In the beginning, as the initial surveys demonstrated, the need was total, since care was nonexistent. In that framework, the AMA standards and the accompanying accreditation process is a reasonable, indeed laudable, attempt to improve health care.

[19]*Standards for Health Services in Correctional Institutions, An Official Report of the American Public Health Association* (Washington, D.C.: American Public Health Association, 1976); *Health Care in Correctional Institutions, Prescriptive Package* (Washington, D.C.: Law Enforcement Assistance Administration, U.S. Department of Justice, 1975).

However, opting for one side, in the radical disjunction of interest between prisoners and their keepers, the AMA program allies itself entirely with the custodians. It recognizes and uses the concepts of direct and secondary benefit to administrative personnel from participation in improving health care; it works as a part of the system. It eschews confrontation with basic prison conditions. Thus, for example, the decision was made in the process of developing the standards to eliminate environmental health issues such as food, sanitation, and overcrowding from the purview of the standards; the ostensible reason was that these areas are covered by other sets of correctional standards. An alternate proposed rationale is that insistence on environmental health standards would make consensus medical standards impossible. Only by limiting the definition of health could the AMA standards pretend to address health needs.

The preface of the 1979 edition of the standards states that

> Accreditation means professional and public recognition of good performance; accreditation through standards implementation, based upon success of other fields, is the foundation for professionalization and the public's recognition of good performance; accreditation through standards implementation, based upon success of other fields, is the foundation for professionalization and the public's recognition of criminal justice medicine.[20]

The standards clearly meet the needs of prison health professionals. Do they meet the needs of inmates?

The latest set of the AMA standards isolates 69 elements that are necessary in an effective prison health care delivery system. It divides the standards into six sections, including standards governing administrative issues, personnel, care and treatment, pharmaceuticals, health records, and medical–legal issues.

---

[20]*Standards for Health Services in Jails, AMA Program to Improve Medical Care and Health Services in Correctional Institutions* (Chicago: AMA Division of Medical Practice, July 1979), preface p. i.

(See Appendix A on page 229 for a listing of essential and important standards.)

It would be foolish to state that a jail which previously provided no medical care could not be vastly improved by the implementation of the AMA standards; clearly the jump from no service to any service will improve the care available to those incarcerated. Implementation of the standards will clearly facilitate the baseline delivery of care, which should prevent unnecessary deaths, contain communicable disease, deal with acute illness and trauma, and prevent much suffering. It must be noted, however, that there is often likely to be a gap between the effect of the implementation of the standards, many of which are merely paper requirements (or requirements for paper, i.e., written procedures and protocols) and the actual achievement of care that is even minimally adequate technically as judged by a community standard.

Thus a medically accredited institution may in fact meet the medical needs (those objective and professionally determined baseline requirements) of inmates. However, it certainly will not meet the articulated health wants and desires of inmates. Nor may it meet those medical needs that may conflict with administrative desire or convenience or that may grow out of the process of imprisonment itself. Accreditation based on the AMA standards may indeed provide the basis for improved health care capacity. However, the implementation of standards should not constitute proof of the adequacy of health care. Only an independent audit can actually assess the adequacy of care. As with any standards, but especially with the AMA standards (which stress the creation of written guides), there is no necessary link between standards, accreditation, and acceptable quality of care.

The wants and desires (some of which could properly be designated needs) about health care of men and women in prisons and jails—as expressed to staff in sessions organized by the Montefiore Hospital Prison Health Project (Department of Social

Medicine)—go far beyond what the process developed by the AMA envisions. Inmates want a medical service (1) to be available whenever they want it; (2) to be usable for ancillary needs aside from health care (e.g., for getting out of work or for being excused from school or program); (3) to provide immediate remedies for any symptom; (4) to provide reassurance that a given illness or symptom has no long-range or dire consequences; (5) to provide a framework for meeting friends in a more unsupervised setting; (6) to provide the possibility for seeing members of the opposite sex; (7) to provide human contact of a warmer and more supportive sort in institutions in which displays of power and brutality both by other inmates and by guards are the rule; (8) to provide remedies for preexisting conditions for which no care is available on the street (e.g., removal of tattoos or old scars or of tracemarks from arms); (9) to remedy long-standing health problems, such as bad teeth or lack of dentures.

How many of these wants and desires are so critical to the health of inmates that they should be encompassed and addressed by standards designed to meet patient needs? How many can be dismissed as outside of the scope and appropriate ambit of the health system? These questions have never been posed, let alone answered.

For inmates in prison, in the words of one lifer at Sing Sing, "Everything hurts more." As connections to the outside world are severed, the focus naturally shifts to self; as the process of infantilization that accompanies imprisonment progresses, there is a natural inclination to demand help for those unmet needs which preexisted incarceration and are only aggravated by the process itself. There is only the medical staff from whom to demand help. Inmates *need* to be healthy; their survival in prison requires it. Yet for their mental health they need to be free, and it is clear that a prison health service cannot recognize this deep level of need or desire. Thus, how can the demands, requests, and desires of inmates be segregated into those with sufficient objective support in health care theory and those properly disregarded as inappropriate?

The standards do not begin to address the specific medical care desires of inmates; they address the process in the prison and the systems of care. For the health *needs* of inmates, those things *required* for them to be healthy in prison are related both to prior health conditions and life-styles and to prison-generated problems. A special inmate health committee at the Woodbourne Correctional Facility (a medium-security prison in New York State) indicated that inmates' perceptions of their health *needs* (those objective factors) focused on problems in the following areas: (1) drug and alcohol dependence; (2) injuries and trauma (relating to sports and exercise and to attack); (3) nutrition—diet and vitamins, especially related to fears about sexual potency; (4) mental health and stress, especially the stress of imprisonment; (5) sexuality—sexual needs and aggressive sexual attack; (6) chronic disease management—especially for hypertension, diabetes, and cardiovascular disease; (7) seizures and seizure disorders; (8) dental care. These were the areas of health *need* defined by inmates in a facility which, in general, complied with the standards developed by the AMA. These were the areas in which the inmates felt, and independent involved professionals agreed, that health problems existed.

Some of the topics listed above are indeed addressed to some degree by the standards. As an example, standards (no. 149) do specify that detoxification be provided in the jails (the prison standard is identical). The standards state:

> written policy and defined procedures require that *detoxification* from alcohol, *opioids*, stimulants and sedative hypnotic drugs is effected as follows: when performed at the facility it is under medical supervision; and, when not performed in the facility, it is conducted in a hospital or community detoxification center.[21]

---

[21]Ibid., p. 25.

Prison literature indicates that over half of those incarcerated have some, and many have an extensive, history of drug and alcohol use. Addiction is one of the primary concerns of an inmate population. In addition to the practical problems presented by reentry into a society with increasing unemployment which is generally unwilling to hire ex-offenders, those in prison know that the temptations, given the frustrations, to turn to drugs and alcohol again are almost overwhelming. A written procedure designed to prevent death from the process of detoxification is created by the standards; the health problem of drug and alcohol dependency is unnoted, unnoticed, and unaddressed.

As another example, consider sports injuries, a major source of problems in all male institutions and specifically at Woodbourne. There injuries occurred in particularly violent basketball games; during regimens of running on the hot pavement in the prison yards, often without proper sneakers and sometimes without sneakers at all; and through the inappropriate use of weightlifting equipment in the weight room. The resulting injuries are the most serious, continuous set of problems referred to the prison health service. The only comment in the standards relevant to this particular health problem is No. 161, entitled "Exercising"[22] (in the section on Care and Treatment); it is not essential and states:

> Written policy and defined procedures outline a program of exercising and require that each inmate is allowed the daily minimum of one hour of exercise involving large muscle activity, away from the cell on a planned, supervised basis.

As a final example, consider the list of health needs recently composed by a group of women in a newly formed health care committee at Bedford Hills (the Correctional Institution for Women

[22]Ibid., p. 30.

in New York State). The list composed by the inmates indicates that their primary health concerns involved (1) cleanliness and hygiene—keeping person, clothes, and dishes clean when one sink is provided for all and when scouring powder is contraband; (2) diet and nutrition, especially obesity; (3) attacks by other inmates—the mental health problems created by living with "touch-offs," firebugs, and attackers; (4) the stress and pressure that come from doing time; (5) lack of sports and exercise; (6) obstetric and gynecologic problems; (7) family reunions; (8) diabetes, hypertension, and back problems; (9) seizures and asthma; and (10) dental care. In response, the standards provide nonessential items on dental care, pregnancy, nutritional requirements, special diets, exercising, and personal hygiene. These are not wants and desires either inappropriate to or beyond the reasonable capability or role of medicine. The inmate-defined problems describe the health needs of these inmates. In most cases, it is appropriate for professionals to define need, while patients content themselves with defining their wants and desires and with finding those able to accommodate these personal preferences. This schema is less appropriate or perhaps inappropriate to prisons where disregard for the honesty, humanness, and value of the prisoner–patient often leads to a less than adequate definition of need and where the patient possesses no opportunity to obtain medical care appropriate to want or desire. Some prisons do, in fact, permit independent private physician visits; most do not. But even where permitted, the cost and inconvenience of a visit combined with the relative rarity of an inmate having a regular private physician make it the infrequent exception. Thus if medicine is, on its own, to define need it must ground this definition of need in the health problems peculiar to prisoners as understood and experienced by them. The definition of need should recognize the inability to secure independent care for any wants or desires.

Conclusion

The paucity or total lack of service delivery capacity in most prisons and jails has been and continues to be so extreme that the implementation of the AMA standards will most likely, with previously stated caveats, improve the ability of many correctional institutions to deliver care. Once a marginal or baseline level of care has been achieved, however, the exclusion of inmates from the process by which the standards were developed and from any ongoing involvement in monitoring the effective implementation of the standards must necessarily affect the likelihood that the standards will help to provide an adequate response to real inmate needs. In many institutions where health care standards are adequate, the size, overcrowded conditions, and procedural obstinacy of the institution result in the lack of access to care; this negates the best of standards and renders even the most excellent staff ineffective or even impotent.

Jail and prison health standards were developed by cooperating professionals in medicine and corrections to improve the health care given to inmates but also to improve the image of correctional and of health professionals. These are not necessarily incompatible aims. However, given the adversary relationships existing between all correctional officials, most health care professionals, and the inmate population, it is unlikely that medical staff subservient to the correctional administration will effectively assess and respond to the needs of prisoners. The AMA demonstrated, in its "pre–post profile" of early participating jails, that the improvements in both the availability and adequacy of health care occurred in every service category, including the following: an increase from 15 jails where chronic and convalescent care were available per program to 21 sites at the end of year two, where they were not only available but adequate, an increase from 12 to 22 sites providing regular sick call to inmates, an increase from 7 to 21 jails offering detoxification for both alcohol and drug abusers, and an increase from 16 to 23 sites providing special diets to inmates.[23]

In addition to recording increased potential for service delivery, the AMA also screened inmates to see whether improvements that occurred in the health care delivery system had any effect on improving the health status of inmates. The evaluators conclude:

> Thus, on an overall basis it seems clear that the objective measures in the I/PP [Inmate Patient Profile], a health status indicator, documented significant increases over time in the availability and adequacy of health care services in accredited jails, and some significant improvement in the provisionally accredited facilities as well. In addition, the evaluators go on to note that increasingly greater proportions of inmates' abnormalities were being identified and treated in the second year than the first. On a subjective basis, though, inmates in the second year were no more satisfied with the health care delivery systems in their jails than were inmates interviewed the first year.[24]

Given the process of evaluation which demonstrated that the health care delivery systems in accredited jails significantly improved, what accounts for the resolute statements of the inmates affected that the health care remains inadequate and unresponsive? (Although it must be emphasized again that patient satisfaction is not necessarily an adequate method for auditing care— only an independent quality-of-care audit by objective measurements will suffice.)

Reasons for this dissatisfaction may be related to the fact that, even in a facility with improved health care delivery capability, the inmates do not sense that delivery capability meets their real needs because those needs were never adequately as-

[23]Anno and Hornung, "Summary," p. 17.
[24]Ibid., p. 19.

sessed. In addition, the dissatisfaction may not reflect the ability or capability of the medical care staff but rather, as previously mentioned, the cooperation and administrative flexibility of the institutional authorities. Access to care may be defined by medical standards; it can only be implemented by correctional administrators with the cooperation of line officers.

The process by which prison health care standards were developed—by professionals, with little regard for or consultation with the population affected—has produced a set of standards protective of the professions involved, crucial for the health status of inmates, but inappropriate for perceived wants and perhaps real health needs. I would suggest that there are, in addition, four related problems:

1. A lack of commonality of class between those proposing standards and those for whom they are developed
2. The lack of any unity of perception as to the real health needs of the inmate population
3. A disregard, on the part of the professionals, for the feelings, perceptions, and life-style health problems of the population
4. A lack of coordinated consultation between professionals and patients or, more harshly stated, the exclusion of those affected from the process by which the standards were developed

As standards of care become more important in discussions around federally funded health programs, the lessons of the prison health care effort may be useful. The disparity between professional and population served will never, quite obviously, be as great. However, the professional expertise model of delivering health care often has a quite large element of disregard for the patient. As standards are developed for appropriate acute care, for ambulatory care, and for specific groups such as the geriatric population, the mentally ill, and the renal diseased, the lessons provided by the growth of prison health standards may be useful.

The lesson learned may be that it is critical to examine the setting, life-style, and peculiar pressures of various groups before setting standards which define the "needs" of those groups. Alternative access to care, mobility, past economic position, education level, health history, and political power all impinge on the pure medical decision as to the "needs" of patients. Equity demands that these factors be examined, weighed, and corrected in devising a fair and useful system.

Standards, by their nature, must be the result of a process of compromise and consensus. Whereas the usual understanding of these terms indicates a meeting place at some mythical point midway between the interests of the two parties, the reality often dictates—as it did in the instance of setting prison health care standards—the imposition by one side (the more powerful and organized) of its perception of interest. As the setting of medical standards, therefore, reflects the needs of patients through the prism of power relationships, those standards may come to move gradually away from the community concept of an acceptable quality of care. Needless to say, the discrepancy in political power, status, and societal acceptance will never be as great for any other group as it is for prisoners. However, as we come to the process of setting standards for the poor and for the elderly, for the migrant worker and the nonunionized factory employee, the quality of those standards must be subjected to special scrutiny.

4

Arthur L. Caplan

How Should Values Count in the Allocation of New Technologies in Health Care?

I

A few years ago Dr. Howard Hiatt, Dean of the Harvard School of Public Health, wrote a provocative article entitled "Protecting the Medical Commons: Who Is Responsible?"[1] Dr. Hiatt noted that as the costs of medical therapy—in terms of time, money and manpower—continue to rise, physicians, health planners, policy analysts, and the general public are faced with a terrible dilemma: how should the finite resources available for health care in American society be allocated? Dr. Hiatt argued that the medical profession must take the responsibility for evaluating expensive new medical technologies and techniques prior to their being made generally available to consumers. His view is that the medical profession should be able to regulate the supply of medical

---

[1]H. H. Hiatt, "Protecting the Medical Commons: Who Is Responsible?" *New England Journal of Medicine*, CCXCIII (1975), 235–40.

Arthur L. Caplan ● Associate for the Humanities, The Hastings Center, Institute of Society, Ethics and the Life Sciences, Hastings-on-Hudson, New York 10706.

services and technologies as a means of controlling the rapidly rising costs of health care. The numerous cases of expensive, ineffective, and ineffectual therapies scattered throughout the history of medical care provide solid empirical grounds for the policy Hiatt suggested.

Unfortunately, technological evolution in medicine is not readily amenable to the type of efficacy testing Hiatt suggests. The steady flow of new technologies, refinements of existing technologies, and resuscitations of old technologies make efficacy testing an enormously difficult affair. The number of drugs, devices, and procedures utilized in medical care today boggles the minds of even the most cost-conscious and quantitatively skilled analysts.

Moreover, the problems surrounding the allocation of medical resources are more complex than matters of supply efficacy. Of course it is reasonable to demand that medical therapies work and work well before they are utilized in actual medical care. But how will efficacy be demonstrated—by what techniques, with what degree of reliability, upon whom, by whom? Who possesses the requisite time, skill, and expertise to carry out efficacy testing— physicians, economists, medical consumers, the government? Furthermore, what values will be utilized in the determination of efficacy—patient needs, patient desires, physician needs, physician desires, potential patient needs, potential patient desires, industry's needs, government's needs, and so on? And what values will be utilized in assessing efficacy—efficiency, justice, desert, benefit, success, and so on?

Questions such as these concerning the estimation and evaluation of efficacy are all too familiar to the hordes of epidemiologists, public health officials, bureaucrats, economists, ethicists, and consumer advocates who have attempted to locate techniques and procedures for providing appropriate answers. The solutions that have been proposed are no longer couched in the mysterious dialect of health planners and analysts. The language of random clinical trials, retrospective studies, cost/benefit analysis, and technology assessment has become part of the common vernacular in legislatures, newspapers, and television programs.

The development of new analytical procedures, new government agencies, and new experts in the health care sector has been fueled by a single overriding concern—cost containment.[2] This concern is not unique to health care but it is, perhaps, more blatantly in evidence there than in other areas involving enormous expenditures of public and private monies. Health care in general and new health care technologies in particular have been allocated during the past decade against a backdrop of cost concerns. Efficacy has always been a concern in medicine, but the preoccupation with rising costs has turned this concern into an obsession.

The quantification of values in the health care sector is both a cause and an effect. The Januslike status of the various analytical techniques that can be lumped under this heading has had a peculiar effect on issues of allocation. Quantification techniques have become the vehicle for generating a crisis atmosphere in medicine. Talk of escalating costs and scarcity has set the stage for discussions of triage concerning the medical commons. At the same time, these same quantification techniques are expected to provide the solutions to the very problems they have identified. This is especially so in that part of medicine utilizing new technologies; that is, the allocation of new drugs, devices, and procedures is to be guided by various quantitative analytical techniques. The development and allocation of CAT-scan devices, artificial hearts, artificial joints, electronic fetal monitoring devices, amniocentesis, mammography, and new vaccines are to be

[2]A. M. B. Golding and D. Tosey, "The Cost of High-Technology Medicine," *The Lancet*, 1980, 195–97; and W. J. McNerney, "Control of Health-Care Costs in the 1980s," *New England Journal of Medicine*, CCCIII (1980), 1088–95.

both inspired and governed by the calculations and quantifica-
tions of value that various experts can and do provide.

II

The purveyors of quantitative techniques have not only defined the problem regarding new technologies in health care
(rising costs) but have also been bold enough to claim that they
can provide the means by which this problem can be solved (cost/
benefit analyses and technology assessment). Numerous government reports on a variety of technologies show the influence and
importance of cost/benefit analysis and technology assessment in
guiding federal policy in the allocation of monies for research,
development, demonstrations, and reimbursement regarding
health technologies.[3] Those federal government agencies—such
as the Food and Drug Administration; the Office of Technology
Assessment; and the Office of Health Research, Statistics, and
Technology—which are active in the assessment and evaluation
of new technologies in health care rely heavily upon cost/benefit
and technology assessment techniques in carrying out their
mandates.

The federal government is not alone in its reliance on these
techniques to solve problems of cost containment and allocation.
Some years ago the National Academy of Engineering issued
guidelines, under the aegis of its Committee on Public Engineering Policy, which are quite explicit about the modes of analysis to be utilized in the planning and assessment of technology:

[3]National Center for Health Services Research, *Medical Technology*, DHEW
Publication No. 79-3254 (1979); National Academy of Sciences, *Assessing Biomedical
Technologies* (Washington, D.C.: 1975); Office of Technology Assessment, *As-
sessing the Efficacy and Safety of Medical Technologies* (Washington, D.C.: U.S.
Government Printing Office, 1978).

1. Identify and refine the subject to be assessed.
2. Delineate the scope of the assessment and develop a data base.
3. Identify alternative strategies to solve the selected problems with the technology under assessment.
4. Identify the parties affected by the selected problems and the technology.
5. Identify the impacts on the affected parties.
6. Valuate or measure the impacts.
7. Compare the pros and cons of alternative strategies.[4]

These recommendations make clear the key steps in technology assessment. They also reveal cost/benefit analyses to be a part of the broader technique of technology assessment, since the last three steps involve the determination of measures of value. There is no doubt that numerous federal policies toward new technologies in medicine have been guided by precisely the type of recipe described in the academy's report.

III

It is important to realize that the crisis of cost regarding new medical technologies has been defined by many of the same people who claim to have techniques and methods for bringing about the solution to the crisis. For example, it is often claimed that the costs of reimbursing dialysis treatment and transplantation for persons suffering from end-stage renal disease (ESRD) are out of control. ESRD payments from Medicaid and Medicare now total well over $1 billion, yet the program serves only 50,000

---

[4]Report of the Committee on Public Engineering Policy, *A Study of Technology Assessment*, (Washington, D.C.: National Academy of Engineering, 1969), 25–26.

individuals. While ESRD patients constitute 0.2% of the total
Medicare population, they account for 5% of all Medicare Part
B expenditures. In the past 10 years, the costs of the program
have increased tenfold.[5]

Despite the size of and rapid increase in payments for ESRD,
recent studies have noted that the program delivers high-quality
therapy to people who otherwise would not have received it.
Moreover, when constant, noninflated dollars are used in computation, much of the rapid increase in government reimbursements can be seen as a function of the general inflation in prices
that has taken place in the economy over the past decade.[6] Thus,
the question of whether this program or other expenditures on
new technologies demand cost containment is not as straightforward as it might appear to be on first inspection. The determination of the need for quantification techniques to rein in rapidly
rising costs revolves around a number of subtle value questions
concerning the definition of *cost* and, more importantly, *too costly*.

The usual technique for quantifying and assessing the information relevant to problems concerning rapidly escalating costs
is cost/benefit analysis. This rubric covers a variety of approaches
to the analysis of cost, including cost-effectiveness analysis and
cost/benefit analysis. Cost-effectiveness methodology attempts to
assess the efficiency with which resources are being applied to
achieve a desired benefit. In cost/benefit analysis, the goal is to
develop a single measure of net value (usually monetary) in light

[5]G. B. Kolata, "Dialysis after Nearly a Decade," *Science*, CCVIII (1980), 473–
76. Also, A. L. Caplan, "Kidneys, Ethics, and Politics: Policy Lessons of the
ESRD Experience," *Journal of Health, Politics, Policy and Law*, VI (1980), 488–
503.

[6]R. A. Rettig, *Implementing the End-Stage Renal Disease Program of Medicare*,
(Santa Monica, Calif.: Rand, 1980), pp. 5–8.

of which a comparative assessment of technology options can be made.[7]

IV

Attempts to quantify values so as to allow a more rational allocation of monies and expenditures of resources have not lacked for critics. Many commentators have noted that cost/benefit approaches to the assessment of technology are based upon flawed assumptions about the amenability of values to quantitative analysis. Criticisms of cost/benefit approaches to solving the riddles of costs and allocation fall roughly into two categories, computational and moral.

Critics of cost/benefit analyses are fond of pointing out the futility involved in attempting to calculate the incalculable.[8] Consider some of the factors involved in a cost/benefit analysis of the various available treatment modalities for renal failure. How is it possible to quantify such ineffable values as a fear of becoming dependent on a machine or the freedom to take a vacation? Attempts to quantify such values in dollars, rankings, or scales seem vain. Moreover, when such values *are* measured, critics note that the resulting calculation is likely to reflect the preferences of the calculator more closely than those of anyone else.

[7]M. C. Weinstein and W. B. Stason, "Foundations of Cost-Effectiveness Analysis for Health and Medical Practices," *New England Journal of Medicine*, CCXCIX (1977), pp. 716–21; and E. J. Mishan, *Benefit-Cost Analysis* (New York: Praeger, 1976).

[8]H. P. Green, "The Risk-Benefit Calculus in Safety Determinations," *George Washington Law Review*, XLIII (1975), pp. 791–807; and B. Williams, "A Critique of Utilitarianism," *Utilitarianism For and Against*, edited by J. J. C. Smart and B. Williams (Cambridge, England: Cambridge University Press, 1973), pp. 77–155.

Other objections to cost/benefit computational techniques revolve around thorny issues of what exactly should be counted as a cost, a benefit, a good, and a consequence of a given policy or therapeutic regimen. How should a time scale be selected in doing cost/benefit analyses? And what degrees of reliability and accuracy should govern cost/benefit calculations? Should we trust the judgments of those doing the computations, or do we have to rely on the opinions of others? And if we require the participation of all those who are affected by a policy or regimen—so as to guarantee an equal hearing for the values of all concerned— of what benefit is the calculation in the first place?[9]

Such criticisms and objections to various efforts to quantify values in the area of medical technology are by now old hat. The economist or policy analyst has heard them all before and is unlikely to be much moved by their force. Choices must be made and, given the severity of the cost problem, the risks of missing a bizarre value or forcing an especially unruly value into a simple taxonomic category are, proponents of quantitative techniques argue, outweighed by the clarity and insights the quantification of values can bring to complex problems such as the allocation of a new medical technology. Ineffability is not likely to carry great weight in a climate where a large number of dollars hang in the balance.

There is, however, a different type of criticism that can be brought to bear against cost/benefit solutions to health technology problems. While most critics focus on in-principle computational difficulties facing the purveyors of cost/benefit analyses, some commentators have observed that the primary problem with the quantification of values is that they represent an illegitimate res-

---

[9]A. MacIntyre, "Utilitarianism and Cost-Benefit Analysis," *Values in the Electric Power Industry*, edited by K. Sayre (Notre Dame, Ind.: University of Notre Dame Press, 1977); M. Sagoff, "Economic Theory and Environmental Law," *Michigan Law Review*, LXXIX (June, 1981), 1393–1419.

olution of a legitimate moral issue. Cost/benefit analyses in health care are acknowledged by critics as well as proponents of these methods to be exclusively concerned with the consequences of action and policy. This concern, however, represents a moral choice—that utilitarianism is the correct moral point of view for resolving questions of allocation.

This choice of moral outlook requires a justification that is rarely forthcoming from those who make it. Those who reject utilitarianism in all its various guises are unlikely to be persuaded by the elegance and power of computational methods and quantitative techniques. For example, those who believe in a basic right of all persons to adequate health care will not be much moved by talk of cost, benefit, or social good. Physicians who believe that their first and only moral duty is to serve their patients' welfare do not practice medicine in light of utilitarian concerns for the public interest, the general good, or the commonweal. On this moral view, those who need renal dialysis are entitled to renal dialysis—come quantitative hell or high water. The quantification of value is more than a calculation of costs and benefits. Often it is ideology masquerading as a moral point of view.[10] Since alternative points of view about what is fair, just, equitable, and right do exist, the calculations provided by cost/benefit analyses are only as valuable as the arguments in favor of the moral position that motivates their computation. Ultimately, the quantification of values (as in cost/benefit analyses of policy options in health care) is only as convincing as the arguments that can be mustered for a totally utilitarian view of mo-

[10]L. H. Tribe, "Technology Assessment and the Fourth Discontinuity: The Limits of Instrumental Rationality," *Southern California Law Review*, XLVI (1973), 617–60. See also T. C. Schelling, "Analytical Methods and the Ethics of Policy," *Ethics in Hard Times*, edited by A. L. Caplan and D. Callahan (New York: Plenum Press, 1981); and John Arras, "Health Care Vouchers and the Rhetoric of Equity," *Hastings Center Report*, XI (August, 1981), 29–39.

rality. The fundamental ineffability confronting those who, in response to the hard choices posed by new medical technologies, might wish to quantify values is the determination of why such an approach is the best solution to genuine moral perplexity.

V

There can be no doubt that moral choices haunt the process of quantifying values at every stage in the analysis of new technologies in health care. Decisions must be made and defended as to the need and rationale for quantification at a particular time, the modes of calculation that will be used, and the desirability of consequentialist solutions to the problems that are posed.

There is, however, yet another problem that stands in the way of the application of quantitative cost/benefit techniques to policy problems in the area of medical technology. Not only is the utility of quantification cast in doubt by failures to justify properly the legitimacy of purported problems and their solutions, but difficulties arise in analyzing and formulating policies about technologies in an area where very little is known about their development and evolution.

Policy analysts and planners use the terms *innovation* and *dissemination* to describe the processes by which technologies evolve from bright ideas to commercial products. But when one looks to the field of medical technology, very little can be found as to either the patterns of evolution characteristic of technological change in this area or the mechanisms governing these patterns. The absence of detailed case histories of technological evolution in medicine—much less of theories of technological change— is particularly troublesome in assessing the adequacy of the answers provided by cost/benefit analysts and other policy planners to questions of allocation and distribution in medicine. The fact that technologies in medicine are subject to constant change, refinement, and alteration makes them particularly difficult targets for policy analysis. Questions of how best to allocate, pay for, and market new technologies in medicine require not only moral decisions as to what constitute legitimate computational techniques but also empirical and theoretical insight into technological evolution. Perhaps the easiest way to illustrate the indispensability of a theoretical understanding of technological evolution for any and all value decisions in medicine is to examine a specific case where the lack of theory has had deleterious consequences for policy. Hemodialysis provides an example of the difficulties involved in making policy choices and resource allocations in the domain of medical technology.

VI

It is important to realize that a significant mythology has somehow arisen about the history, costs, and funding of ESRD. Some of the most common myths are the following:

1. The large increase in the number of people in America receiving renal dialysis therapy during the 1970s is attributable *solely* to the availability of federal funding for reimbursing the cost of dialysis.[11]

---

[11]As Renee Fox, among many authors, has argued, "Dialysis became increasingly available to a larger number of people even before the passage of the Public Law, but the extensive financial coverage that the legislation made possible is the major factor that accounts for the dramatic change in accessibility of dialysis." *Essays in Medical Sociology* (New York: Wiley, 1979), p. 139.

2. The allocation of the supply[12] of renal dialysis and transplants is contingent upon the availability of funds to reimburse medical professionals for these services.
3. Countries with socialized systems of medical care never
   did and do not now exclude people in need from the
   supply of treatments for renal failure.
4. People's needs determine the nature of the health care
   supply that is available.
5. The current cost of the supply for those in need due to
   renal failure is simply a result of the need rising to meet
   the availability of federal funds to pay the costs.[13]

The easiest way to debunk these elements of the mythology
surrounding ESRD is to review the history of the technology and
its funding. If some headway can be made in this enterprise, a
more realistic and reasonable assessment can then be made of
the ESRD program and its lessons for health policy in general
and the analysis of value choices in health care in particular.

VII

One of the most puzzling gaps in the extant normative analyses of the ESRD program is the lack of attention to the key role
of technological evolution in micro- and macroallocative deci-

---

[12]*Health care supply* is any mode of medical therapy for meeting a health care
need. Health care needs are assessments by health care professionals of the
means required to attain or maintain a state of health for a given person. When
a health care supply exists for meeting a need, the need can be said to be
actionable. *Health care wants* involve the subjective desires of individuals for
a health care supply. The doctor–patient relationship can usefully be conceptualized as a process of negotiation between doctor and patient over whether
a particular health care supply is a need and is actionable. See Mark Siegler's
essay in this volume for an analysis of the specifics of doctor–patient negotiations.
[13]D. Rennie, "Home Dialysis and the Costs of Uremia," *New England Journal
of Medicine*, CCXCVIII (1978), 399–400.

sions. As new medical technologies appear and evolve, the criteria for allocating them also shift and evolve. The history of chronic renal dialysis therapy contains at least four key stages of development: invention, advertising, acceptance, and mastery. Allocation policies cannot be understood or analyzed unless they are placed in the context of this evolutionary sequence, since there is a direct relationship between technological evolution and value choice in medicine.

Invention

Artificial kidney machines capable of removing waste materials from blood evolved after World War II. By 1950 several American medical centers had artificial kidney machines[14] that were used to "rest" the kidneys of diseased patients in the hope this would allow malfunctioning kidneys to regain their normal function. The technological problems confronting those interested in using a mechanical kidney to treat chronic renal failure involved access to the machine, not the machine itself.

The use of the artificial kidney machine could be accomplished only by the insertion of tubes or cannulas into an artery and a vein. Each treatment required a new artery and vein, since previously used sites could not be reused. Since each treatment destroyed an accessible artery and vein, physicians using the artificial kidney quickly ran out of usable sites for gaining access to a patient's circulation. Thus, artificial kidneys could be used only to treat acute cases of renal failure. Chronic filtration of the blood was impossible due to the problem of access.

This problem remained unsolved until the invention of the arteriovenous shunt by Belding Scribner of the University of Washington in 1959. As Richard Rettig has correctly noted, "This

[14]Richard A. Rettig, "Health Care Technology: Lessons Learned from the End-Stage Renal Disease Experience," *The Rand Paper Series*, P-5820 (November, 1976), 1–36.

was the critical technological invention that ushered in the use
of the artificial kidney to maintain the lives of those suffering
from chronic kidney failure."[15]

Scribner realized[16] that by placing a permanent tube or shunt
between an accessible artery and vein, blood circulation to these
vessels could be maintained while permitting continuous access
to the general circulation. The subcutaneous shunt could simply
be removed for short periods of time and replaced by a shunt
leading to the kidney machine. By permanently "short-circuiting"
the circulation in an artery and vein through a shunt, a permanent
access site could be kept in place in a chronically ill person.

Scribner's shunt changed the nature of medical intervention
for renal failure. What had formerly been only an acute therapy
for both acute and chronic renal failure now became a potential
chronic therapy for cases of chronic[17] disability.

Advertising

Having devised the shunt, Scribner spent the next three
years, from 1959 to 1962, disseminating his new invention to the
medical community. He made presentations at various medical
society meetings and brought samples of his shunt with him to
demonstrate to interested colleagues.[18] A steady procession of
young physicians came to Seattle from around the country to
study Scribner's technique.[19]

[15]Ibid., p. 4.
[16]As reported in R. C. Fox and J. P. Swazey, *The Courage to Fail*, 2nd. ed.
(Chicago: University of Chicago Press, 1978).
[17]For more on the history of Scribner's shunt, see J. W. Czaczkes and A. Kaplan
De-Nour, *Chronic Hemodialysis as a Way of Life* (New York: Brunner/Mazel,
1978), chap. 2.
[18]Rettig, "Health Care Technology," pp. 11–13.
[19]Richard Rettig, "Valuing Lives: The Policy Debate on Patient Care Financing
For Victims of End-Stage Renal Disease," *Rand Paper Series* P-5672 (March,
1976), 20–21.

One of the most active participants in this form of advertising the new shunt technology was the hospital system of the Veterans Administration. In 1963 the VA announced a program for establishing dialysis centers in 30 VA hospitals around the country.[20] This was a critical step in the course of disseminating renal dialysis treatment for chronic renal failure, since many of the people in renal medicine received training in VA hospitals and learned to perform dialytic therapy in the setting of long-term chronic care institutions. Since the VA population is primarily institution-based, it was reasonable for the VA to ask for funds for the construction of renal dialysis units in VA hospitals. While some commentators have suggested that the current emphasis on center-based dialysis is a result of more lucrative federal reimbursement rates, this emphasis actually dates back to the first involvement of VA hospitals with dialysis.

By 1968 about 1,000 people were receiving long-term renal dialysis in America.[21] A number of people were trained or in training to learn to administer chronic dialysis. At this time it was also realized that thousands of others were not receiving dialysis but might benefit from this treatment.

It was roughly at this time that the first of what eventually became a torrent of articles was published on the normative issues involved in allocating renal dialysis machines to particular individuals.[22] It is important to note that these articles were written at a time when dialysis therapy was still in its infancy and when very few people had any familiarity with the technique.

[20]Ibid., pp. 30–31.

[21]Louise B. Russell, *Technology in Hospitals* (Washington, D.C.: Brookings, 1979), p. 111.

[22]See, for example, S. Alexander, "They Decide Who Lives, Who Dies," *Life*, Nov. 9, 1962, pp. 100–4; H. S. Abram and W. Wadlington, "Selection of Patients for Artificial and Transplanted Organs," *Annals of Internal Medicine*, LIX (1968), 615–20; H. K. Beecher, "Scarce Resources and Medical Advancement," *Daedalus*, XCVIII (1969), 275–313; N. Rescher, "The Allocation of Exotic Medical Lifesaving Therapy," *Ethics*, LXXIX (1969), 173–86.

The short period of time involved from Scribner's invention to the first articles on the ethics of microallocation is significant, since this entire period was one in which renal dialysis (and transplantation) had a rather ambiguous status in the eyes of the medical profession. Some physicians were convinced that dialysis for chronic renal failure was a legitimate medical therapy. Others remained unconvinced and adopted this attitude that dialysis and transplantation were better understood as experimental proce- dures.[23] Scribner had obtained good results using his shunt with his patients during this period, but physicians at other centers had encountered problems in matching his favorable morbidity and mortality rates. The art of carrying out renal dialysis was slow to evolve, due partly to the small number of people capable of carrying out dialysis and, surprisingly, partly to the success obtained initially by Scribner himself. This initial success made dialysis appear to be more a proven therapy than an experimental procedure. Research grants were difficult to obtain for a proce- dure that seemed to involve the provision of a supply to people in need.[24]

Acceptance

The debate over the experimental status of renal dialysis was not "officially"[25] settled until 1967. The Committee on Chronic Kidney Disease, an influential government commission, headed by Dr. C. W. Gottschalk, issued a report which stated:

> The Committee believes that transplantation and dialysis tech- niques are sufficiently perfected at present to warrant launching a national treatment program and urges this course of action. . . .

---

[23]Rettig, "Valuing Lives," pp. 13–16.
[24]Rettig, "Valuing Lives," pp. 24–25.
[25]Rettig uses this term to describe the decision of the Gottschalk Committee. "Valuing Lives," p. 16.

> Approximately 5,000 patients with chronic uremia died in fiscal
> year 1967 because of a lack of adequate treatment facilities and by
> 1973, when treatment capabilities may meet demand, a minimum
> of 24,000 additional medically suitable patients will have died with-
> out the opportunity for treatment.[26]

In the eyes of many in the medical profession, chronic renal dialysis remained only an interesting experimental procedure until 1967.

One other factor which played a key role in the medical profession's skeptical attitude toward dialysis during the 1960s was that dialysis was in direct competition with other techniques for treating renal failure. Renal transplantation, from living and cadaver donors, held out great promise as a less costly[27] and less disruptive treatment. While immunologic rejection posed great difficulties for transplant proponents, many believed that this problem could be solved and that a transplant would be far more attractive to potential patients than a long course of weekly dialysis sessions.

As a consequence of its novelty, chronic dialysis, was not only viewed as experimental but also as only one of a number of possible techniques for treating renal failure.[28] Renal dialysis was in the eyes of many physicians competing with live and cadaver transplantation for the same therapeutic niche.

---

[26]U.S. Bureau of the Budget, *Report of the Committee on Chronic Kidney Disease* (Washington, D.C.: U.S. Government Printing Office, September, 1967), pp. 2–4.

[27]H. F. Klarman, J. O. Francis, and G. D. Rosenthal, "Cost Effectiveness Analysis Applied to the Treatment of Chronic Renal Disease," *Medical Care*, VI (1968), 48–54.

[28]In addition to dialysis in a medical center and renal transplants, possible alternative treatments included home dialysis, peritoneal dialysis, and dietary management. See E. A. Friedman *et al.*, "Pragmatic Realities in Uremia Therapy," *New England Journal of Medicine*, CCDCVIII (1978), 368–371; and Russell, *Technology in Hospitals*, Appendix D.

Mastery

The fourth and last stage in the evolution and development of renal dialysis took place during the period from 1968 to about 1977. During this period the iatrogenic effects of chronic renal dialysis were observed and techniques developed to master them. While dialysis had been employed since the early 1950s as a temporary procedure for people in acute renal failure, the technique had not been used as a treatment for *chronic* renal failure. During the period from 1968 to 1977 enough patient-hours were accumulated on dialysis machines to detect a number of complications and side effects directly attributable to chronic dialysis. Imbalances in metabolites, anemia, hepatitis, cardiovascular anomalies, neuropathy, hypertension, psychiatric problems, and osteodystrophy all emerged as problems directly attributable to chronic renal dialysis.[29]

Various techniques for coping with these problems evolved, ranging from alternating the amount of time on and frequency of dialysis to providing supplementary salts and metabolites to those receiving dialysis.[30] It was only when physicians had accumulated enough experience with chronic dialysis that they were able to diagnose and manage its dangerous side effects. Mastery of the technique was delayed, since there were no data on the iatrogenic effects of *chronic* renal dialysis.

The differences between the acceptance and mastery stages in the evolution of renal dialysis are worth emphasizing. At the end of the third stage, in 1968, Scribner's shunt had gained acceptance among the medical community. There were a small number of trained medical personnel and dialysis centers, in the VA hospitals and elsewhere, to provide dialysis. Approximately

[29]Thomas Manis and Eli A. Friedman, "Dialytic Therapy for Irreversible Uremia," *New England Journal of Medicine*, CCCI (1979), 1321–28.
[30]Ibid., pp. 1323–26.

1,000 persons were receiving dialysis, although few had been in dialysis for more than five years.

By 1977, some 35,000 people were receiving dialysis in the United States; many of them had been on dialysis for 10 years or more.[31] A large number of iatrogenic side effects of chronic dialysis had been identified and techniques had been developed to manage them.

A significant amount of time was needed to move from the stage where chronic dialysis was accepted as a legitimate therapy by the medical profession to the stage at which the medical profession could legitimately be said to have mastered its technique. These stages are crucial for understanding the normative criteria that influenced patient selection during the history of renal dialysis therapy.

VIII

Between 1959 and 1977, the pool of people receiving dialysis for chronic renal failure expanded at a rapid rate, as did the number of personnel prepared to offer dialysis and the number of sites at which dialysis could be obtained.

Perhaps the most marked shift in the composition of the recipient pool for chronic dialysis in the United States took place between the period of "acceptance" of the technique in the late 1960s and "mastery" of the technique in the late 1970s. In the late 1960s, the majority of dialysis recipients were young (25 to 45), middle-class people with no other illnesses. In the words of one physician, "We had what was in many ways an idealized population. A large fraction of the patients were living in a pro-

---

[31]Russell, *Technology in Hospitals*, p. 111. In 1979, some 46,000 patients were receiving dialysis. See Kolata, "Dialysis," p. 473.

ductive period of their lives. They were young and had little else wrong with them."[32]

By the late 1970s the patient pool had shifted considerably. Recipients were often either much older or much younger than in the 1960s. Age and complicating diseases, such as diabetes or alcoholism, were rarely invoked as contraindications for chronic dialysis. Many more poor and minority persons received dialysis care.[33]

The shift in the composition of the patient population for dialysis is sometimes attributed to the ethical biases of physicians in the selection of dialysis recipients and to the availability of funds for chronic dialysis after 1972.[34] But the history of renal dialysis therapy clearly reveals a number of other factors at work in influencing the composition of the patient pool over the years. Far fewer centers and trained personnel existed in the 1960s. Physicians in the 1960s had not fully mastered the technique of chronic dialysis, having no experience with its possible side effects. And chronic renal dialysis was a treatment in competition with other treatments for renal failure during much of the 1960s. In such circumstances the desire of those working with chronic dialysis, both for success as compared to alternative therapies and for mastery over the complications of chronic dialysis, greatly influenced the type of person selected for dialysis in 1967 and 1977. In 1967 physicians wanted "healthy" patients, since a good track record and a "clean" data sample were essential to both

[32]As quoted in ibid., p. 473.
[33]Ibid., p. 474.
[34]Rescher, "Allocation of Therapy." Also, Paul Ramsey, *The Patient As Person* (New Haven, Conn.: University Press, Yale 1970); J. Childress, "Who Shall Live When Not All Can Live?" *Soundings*, XLIII, (1970), 339–62; L. R. Adams, "Medical Coverage For Chronic Renal Disease: Policy Implications," *Health and Social Work*, III (1978), 41–53; M. D. Basson, "Choosing among Candidates for Scarce Medical Resources," *Journal of Medicine and Philosophy*, IV (1979), 313–33.

competitive success and technical mastery. In 1977 neither of
these concerns carried as much weight.

IX

In 1972 Congress passed Public Law 92-603 as an amendment to the Social Security Act. Under this law Medicare coverage was extended to those under 65 suffering from ESRD.

The portion of the law concerning ESRD was passed with
little debate or analysis. Few cost estimates were obtained and
no study of possible supply options was undertaken. The highlight
of the legislative process prior to the passage of the law was the
dialysis of the vice-president of the National Association of Patients on Hemodialysis and Transplantation before the House
Ways and Means Committee in November 1971. The actual
amendment was passed after 30 minutes of debate in the Senate
and 10 minutes in the House in October 1972.[35]

The need for therapy for ESRD seemed clear to the legislators. All that stood between the 24,000 untreated people cited
in the Gottschalk Report and life was money. Renal patients and
physicians wanted the law passed and lobbied for it. In addition,
the ESRD program was only an amendment tacked onto the much
larger Medicare/Medicaid program. Thus, the ESRD program
passed very quickly.

The bill provided money for the reimbursement of renal
therapy to "kidney disease centers" which met minimal standards
for utilization and admission. Physicians were paid a fixed fee per
month for a kidney patient seen in a center, a lower fee for
patients treated at home. Reimbursement fees were also set for

[35]Fox and Swazey, *Essays*, pp. 346–51.

overhead center costs. No limits were set on total reimbursement expenditures for the ESRD program.[36]

One immediate effect of the bill was to encourage the creation of dialysis centers both in and out of medical centers. With reimbursement available at maximum rates for center dialysis, efforts to encourage home dialysis and self-dialysis waned. In 1972, 40% of all patients were dialyzed in their homes. This percentage fell to 15% by 1978.[37]

X

The British experience with ESRD has differed to some extent from the American. Britain has had a national health insurance scheme in place since 1946. However, confronted by the great costs involved in renal therapy, the Department of Health and Social Security took the unusual step of setting a cap on the total amount of money available to treat renal failure. In the words of their 1971 report:

> We actually set aside a sum of money which we told the Hospital
> Boards should be spent on dialysis and we determined where it
> should be spent and how much should be spent. At this time this
> was a great change from our normal method of control and indeed
> we have hardly repeated it since.[38]

This cap of total expenditures had the effect of increasing the percentage of patients in Britain on home as opposed to center dialysis. In 1976, 66% of all patients in the United Kingdom were receiving home dialysis.[39]

[36]Rennie, "Home Dialysis," p. 399.
[37]Robert J. Wineman, "Federal Legislation and Agency Actions Concerning Self-Care Dialysis," *Journal of Dialysis*, II (1978), 103–109.
[38]Quoted in M. H. Cooper, *Rationing Health Care* (New York: Halsted, 1975), p. 92.
[39]*Proceedings of the European Dialysis and Transplant Association*, XIII (Hamburg, Germany: Pitman Medical, 1976), p. 18.

A most interesting aspect of the British experience with ESRD is that despite the availability of governmental funds for ESRD throughout the 1960s and 1970s, the number and composition of the population of patients receiving dialysis and transplants closely parallels the American experience. In the early days of the evolution of dialysis technology, from 1962 to 1966, British physicians were as selective as their American counterparts in placing patients in renal failure on dialysis. Four out of five candidates were rejected. The average patient was middle-aged, male, married, working, and owned his own home.[40] As in America, the small number of trained personnel and the scarcity of dialysis equipment undoubtedly caused the rationing of supply. A large amount of patient need simply was not actionable during the intervention and advertising stages of dialysis development.

The acceptance stage of renal technology showed many parallels as well. Victor Parsons, chief nephrologist at King's College Hospital in London, in commenting about dialysis in the late 1960s, writes:

> Individual desire to go on living or the desire to be treated [for renal failure] was not considered . . . very often the patients were unaware they were up for selection. This enabled the renal units to achieve high survival rates, and quite rightly since in the early stages it was important that the treatment should be seen in its best possible light. To have adopted a totally nonselective policy at the outset would have led the technique into disrepute as being nothing but a technical exercise in the prolongation of a very poor quality of life.[41]

Technological and scientific concerns with demonstrating the superiority, efficacy, and safety of dialysis were as much on the minds of British physicians operating under a socialized system

---

[40]V. Parsons, "The Ethical Challenges of Dialysis and Transplantation," *The Practitioner*, CCXX (1978), 872–77.
[41]Ibid., p. 872.

of health care as they were on the minds of American physicians under a fee-for-service system in the pre-Medicare/Medicaid days.

As the technology of dialysis passed from the stage of acceptance to that of mastery during the 1970s, the pool of dialysis patients in Britain quickly expanded. More centers were built and professional staff trained. The tacitly agreed upon maximum age for dialysis treatment rose from 45 in 1963 to roughly 60 in 1978.[42] However, the financial limits imposed by the cap on overall funding for dialysis, with the resulting emphasis on home dialysis, now discourages British physicians from dialyzing those over 55 and those suffering complicating illnesses such as diabetes or psychological problems.[43]

The patterns of dialysis allocation manifested in the British experience strongly highlight the role of technological evolution in determining the composition of the patient pool. Technological and scientific considerations played just as central a role in microallocation decisions in the early days of dialysis development in the socialized health care system of Britain as they did in the fee-for-service system in the United States.

Further evidence for the role of technological evolution in allocation is provided by the Swedish experience with dialysis. The number and nature of people receiving treatment over the past 20 years also closely parallels that found in the United States despite the availability of public funds. In the 1960s, Swedish

---

[42]Ibid., p. 872.

[43]See Royal College of Physicians Medical Services Study Group, "Deaths From Chronic Renal Failure Under the Age of 50," *British Medical Journal*, CCLXXXIII (July 25, 1981), 283–87, and V. Parsons and P. Lock, "Triage and the Patient with Renal Failure," *Journal of Medical Ethics*, VI (1980), 173–76. In fact, the constraints of money and personnel facing British nephrologists today have caused them to narrow the range of persons deemed in need of or "suitable" for dialysis to the point where many are excluded from treatment who would be dialyzed in the United States. See A. L. Caplan, "Audit in Renal Failure," *British Medical Journal*, CCLXXXIII (September 12, 1981), 727.

physicians were highly selective in admitting people for dialytic therapy. As a recent review of the state of renal therapy in Sweden notes:

> it became a question for nephrologists who had commenced or planned to start long-term dialysis treatment, not only to show that the therapy can prolong life but also that these patients can be rehabilitated, i.e., care for their families and be able to work and pay their taxes. This is in itself remarkable as previously no such criteria had been established to justify the treatment of chronically ill patients.[44]

And, as in the United States and United Kingdom, the shift of renal dialysis from the stage of acceptance in the 1960s to mastery in the 1970s

> has led to a slackening of the previously strict requirements for complete rehabilitation. Nowadays even patients who do not measure up to these requirements—such as the elderly and patients with severe complicating illnesses—are considered for active treatment.[45]

XI

Before returning to the general issues raised at the beginning of this paper, the five popular myths underlying many discussions of the implications of ESRD for health policy deserve some comment, for the history of funding and technology in the area of ESRD is in conflict with all of them.

1. The large increase in the number of people receiving renal dialysis in America is attributable solely to the availability of federal funds for reimbursing the costs of such care.

---

[44]E. Bergsten et al., "A Study of Patients on Chronic Haemodialysis," *Scandinavian Journal of Social Medicine*, Supplement 11 (1977), p. 7.
[45]Ibid., p. 7.

This statement is simply false. The increase in patient numbers is attributable not only to the creation of the ESRD program in 1972 but also to shifts in the status of renal dialysis, from invention to acceptance as a therapy and from acceptance to the mastery of the therapy by the medical profession. The British and Swedish experience with ESRD plainly reveals that factors other than government reimbursement have been at work in expanding the pool of people receiving dialysis.

2. The allocation of the supply of renal dialysis (and transplants) is contingent upon the availability of funds to reimburse medical professionals for these services.

This claim is false, since the supply available for meeting health needs is contingent on much more than money. Scientific and technological concerns affect both the nature of the supply (home dialysis, center dialysis, or transplants) and who gets the supply (young, old, healthy, etc.). The mode of funding affects the degree to which any given person's need is seen as actionable—caps in Britain produce a mode of supply that excludes people over 55 and a definition of need which is far more narrow than that utilized by American physicians.

3. Countries with socialized systems of medical care never did and do not now exclude people in need from the supply of treatments for renal failure.

While this claim is believed by many health planners as well as critics of the American health care system, it is quite false. Rationing existed in Britain and Sweden in a form similar to that which existed in the United States and continues to exist in Britain today.[46]

4. People's needs determine the nature of the health care supply that is available.

This statement is false because it overlooks the role played

---

[46]V. Parsons and P. Lock, "Triage."

by technological evolution in determining the nature and kind of available health care supplies. Technological competition plays a key role in determining the nature of the health care supply. The mode of health care funding also determines supply. Incentives for center dialysis in America have produced a very different supply for renal therapy than that available in Britain.

5. The current cost of the supply for those in need due to renal failure is simply a result of need rising to meet the availability of federal funds to pay the costs.

While the writings of many health policy analysts indicate their credence in this statement,[47] the ESRD experience shows that it is simply not true. The proliferation in the cost of renal dialysis was not due solely to supply rising to meet a windfall of federal dollars.

The high costs involved in the treatment of ESRD can be attributed to the nature and timing of the availability of federal funds. By funding the ESRD program in 1972, the government paid for a technology that was still midway between acceptance and mastery. The cost of 'working the bugs out' of dialysis was paid for under Medicare. The cost of expanding the number of centers and the numbers of trained personnel to staff them was also borne by the United States taxpayer in the form of amortized costs included in treatment fees.

The real policy issue arising from the ESRD program, which myth (5) obscures, is at what point (if ever) should the federal government pay for new technologies in medicine—at the time of invention, acceptance, or mastery?[48]

---

[47]E. G. Knox, "Principles of Allocation of Health Care Resources," *Journal of Epidemiology and Community Health*, XXXII (1978), 309; and Stephen Roberts *et al.*, "Cost-Effective Care of End-Stage Renal Disease: A Billion Dollar Question," *Annals of Internal Medicine*, XCII (1980), 243–48.

[48]John B. McKinlay, "From 'Promising Report' to 'Standard Procedure': Seven Stages in the Career of a Medical Innovation," *Milbank Memorial Fund Quarterly*, LIX (1981), 374–411.

It is not true that the need for dialysis simply expanded. What happened was that the mastery of renal dialysis technology allowed for the reclassification by the medical profession of the particular health needs of various persons from non-actionable to actionable needs.

XII

The real moral issues facing health policy planners is the stance they will adopt toward new and evolving medical therapies. The problem is that our knowledge of technological evolution is so poor that it is hard to classify or analyze the state of particular treatments. Since need and demand are not the sole determinants of cost, our ignorance about the ways in which various modes of medical therapy evolve is a major stumbling block for anticipating the ultimate "cost" of any new medical technology. It is even harder to anticipate the cost of treating medical needs when the evolutionary status of the treatments involved is controversial and the possibility exists that what is untreatable today could be treatable in 5 or 10 years.

There is also an important lesson in the ESRD experience for those concerned with the ethics of health care. Much of the literature on the ethics of microallocation in the area of dialysis and transplant simply misses the mark. By ignoring the history of renal technology and funding, philosophers and theologians have managed to give some very convincing answers to the wrong question. The question is not who should get the kidney machine. In thinking about the normative issues involved in ESRD, the questions are: Who should pay for developing and disseminating new medical therapies, and how can therapeutic and scientific needs best be accommodated in developing any new technology?

XIII

There are important lessons to be learned from the history of hemodialysis therapy for ESRD. In an area such as medical technology one must remember that moral choices concerning allocation are not made in a vacuum. Technological values play a central role in determining the way such choices are resolved. The manner in which various values count in the allocation of medical technologies is determined both by moral choices as to computational and quantitative assessment techniques and by the contingencies of technological development and technological need. As the case of hemodialysis plainly reveals, the values of those supplying the technology do not always overlap with the individual interests of those who might benefit most from receiving the technology.

Most criticisms of efforts to quantify values in the area of technology assessment center around the problems involved in accurately computing fuzzy or peculiar values. The problem of the ineffable is indeed a serious problem for the project of quantifying values. But the most serious problem facing this effort is neither computational nor moral; it is theoretical. We simply do not have available a comprehensive theory of technological evolution upon which to base any sort of valuational analysis—quantitative, intuitive, or other. Without such a theory there is a grave danger that medical technologies will appear and evolve in ways that make their development and allocation inefficient, costly, and unjust. Moreover, if physicians and engineers are to be the gatekeepers of cost and efficacy in the realm of medical technology,[49] we must realize the price we shall pay in terms of the resources allocated for individual medical needs at any given

[49]F. Mosteller, "Innovation and Evaluation," *Science*, CCXI (1981), 881–86.

time. Quantitative values analyses and reliable demonstrations of efficacy will not always work to the optimal benefit of the individual who is sick or diseased. The concerns of the researcher are not those of the therapist or patient. The assessment of technology must be sensitive to these inherent conflicts of interest if it is not to run roughshod over any one of them.

The analysis of the development and evolution of hemodialysis therapy for ESRD may, perhaps, be a first step in the development of a general theory of technological evolution.[50] The role played by competition in filling a particular therapeutic niche—as occurred between hemodialysis, renal transplantation and peritoneal dialysis for treating renal failure—can probably be usefully extended to understand the allocation of other technologies where similar competitive situations obtain. The four stages of development to be found in dialysis technology—invention, advertising, therapy, and mastery—are likely to have analogues in other areas of new medical technology such as the artificial heart. The possession of a formula is not sufficient for allocating scarce new medical technologies; we must be informed and wise as well.

ACKNOWLEDGMENTS

I would like to thank the members of The Hastings Center Project on Ethics and Health Policy for their comments and suggestions on an earlier draft of this paper. I benefited greatly from a variety of comments and suggestions from faculty members at the School of Engineering at the University of Michigan when this paper was given as an invited address.

[50]Judith L. Wagner, "Toward a Research Agenda on Medical Technology," *Medical Technology*, DHEW Publication 79-3254 (Washington, D.C.: National Center for Health Services Research, 1979), pp. 1–12.

5

John Arras

The Neoconservative Health Strategy

VOUCHERS AND THE RHETORIC OF EQUITY

A new medical conservatism has emerged from the health care politics of the last decade. In both style and content, this movement bears little resemblance to the old politics practiced for so many years by the American Medical Association (AMA). The spokesmen of that earlier era tended to be uniformly strident, uncompromising, and fiercely ideological in their defense of the status quo. By contrast, the proponents of the new conservatism are consistently moderate, conciliatory, and pragmatic. Since most of them are university-based scholars rather than physicians, their writing tends to lack that element of intense and often hysterical self-interest that characterized their predecessors' style. The content of their proposals reflects this spirit of reasonableness and accommodation to the modern world. For example, they unabashedly proclaim the need for National Health Insurance (NHI)

An earlier version of this essay was written during my tenure (1979–80) as a Post-Doctoral Fellow at The Hastings Center.

John Arras ● Department of Social Medicine, Montefiore Hospital and Medical Center, Bronx, New York 10467 and Visiting Associate Professor of Philosophy, Barnard College, Columbia University, New York, New York 10027.

in one form or other; they criticize fee-for-services arrangements in favor of prepaid group practices; and they even chide the medical profession for preaching a flinty capitalism while enjoying the fruits of a cushy monopoly. As sociologist Paul Starr wryly notes, the "socialized medicine" of one era has become the corporate reform of the next.[1]

In addition to these striking differences, there are other reasons for dubbing this new force in health politics a "medical neoconservatism." This allusion to the political arena is intentional and appropriate.[2] As described by their most ardent proponent, Irving Kristol, contemporary "neoconservatives" agree on the following three points: (1) they approve of the welfare state but remain critical of the intrusive and paternalistic state; (2) they view the market as the most efficient mechanism for allocating resources and preserving individual freedom; and (3) they espouse traditional notions of equality of opportunity but

[1]Paul Starr, "The Undelivered Health System," *The Public Interest*, Winter, 1976, p. 71.

[2]For an excellent general account of neoconservatism, see Peter Steinfels, *The Neoconservatives: The Men Who Are Changing America's Politics* (New York: Simon & Schuster, 1979). A short list of prominent neoconservative health policy theorists includes Paul Ellwood of Interstudy, a research institute of Minneapolis; Alain Enthoven, an economist at the Stanford Graduate School of Business; Charles Fried, a Harvard law professor; Clark Havighurst, professor of law at Duke; the late Reuben Kessel, formerly of the Graduate School of Business, University of Chicago; and Martin Feldstein, a prominent conservative economist from Harvard. Although Feldstein's views are influential in health policy circles—and would have to be carefully studied in a more comprehensive project— his Major Risk Insurance plan relies so heavily on deductibles and coinsurance that it practically *guarantees* an inequitable outcome for the poor and near-poor. Since equity in health care is the primary concern of this essay, I have chosen to concentrate on those theorists who at least regard the achievement of equity as a serious policy goal. See Martin Feldstein, "A New Approach to National Health Insurance," *The Public Interest*, Spring, 1971, pp. 93–105. A handy anthology of neoconservative writings on health policy has been edited by Cotton M. Lindsay, *New Directions in Public Health Care: A Prescription for the 1980s* (3rd ed.; San Francisco: Institute for Contemporary Studies, 1980).

reject more stringent forms of egalitarianism that insist on "equal shares for everyone."[3] On all three of these counts the medical neoconservatives are in perfect harmony with their political cousins.

It is important to recognize that this movement is not merely an academic fashion. While these academicians naturally lack the enormous clout of the AMA, they are in the vanguard of a growing political movement that is making its influence felt in both the medical establishment and the corridors of political power. Prestigious medical journals have featured articles outlining the new "consumer choice" health strategy,[4] several "procompetition" reform measures were introduced to the ninety-sixth Congress,[5] and, most importantly, some of the most forceful advocates of this new strategy have achieved positions of confidence and power within the Reagan administration. Professor Alain Enthoven, whose important Consumer Choice Health Plan (CCHP) will be discussed at length below, served as adviser on health policy to President-elect Reagan, while legislators Richard Schweiker, David Stockman, and David Durenberger—all authors of procompetition bills—are now (respectively) Secretary of Health and Human Services, Director of the Office of Management and Budget, and chair of the Health Subcommittee of the Senate Finance Committee.[6] This "counterrevolution in health care policy," to use

[3]Kristol's two other criteria—a visceral aversion to the "counterculture" and, in foreign policy, a suspicion of isolationism and détente—are irrelevant to the politics of health care. See Irving Kristol, "What is a Neo-Conservative?" *Newsweek*, Jan. 19, 1976, p. 87; quoted by Steinfels, pp. 53–54.

[4]Alain C. Enthoven, "Consumer-Choice Health Plan," *New England Journal of Medicine*, CCXC (March 23 & 30, 1978), pp. 650–58 and 709–20.

[5]The authors of these bills included Senators David Durenberger (R-Minn.), Richard Schweiker (R.-Pa.), and Representative David Stockman (R.-Mich.).

[6]For a description and discussion of these bills, see Alain Enthoven, "The Competition Strategy: Status and Prospects," *New England Journal of Medicine*, CCXCIII (Jan. 8, 1981), 109–12. For Stockman's views, see his "Rethinking Federal Health Policy: Unshackle the Health Care Consumer," *National Journal*, XI (June 2, 1972).

Stockman's phrase, is thus serious, intelligent, and increasingly influential. Since its essential features are likely to be enacted by the Reagan team, the neoconservatiye health strategy ought to be scrutinized before it becomes policy.

This market-oriented health strategy will, I believe, fail to meet one of its two major objectives: the achievement of a decent standard of equity in the delivery of health seryices. While I also doubt that this strategy will control costs—its primary goal—I shall leave that issue to the economists.[7]

The Causes of Market Failure

The new conservatives' analysis of market failure in health care is based on widely shared premises.[8] The main problems are obviously runaway costs, inflation, and inequity in the delivery of services.

The causes of our nation's soaring health bill—which reached 9% of the gross national product in 1980—are easy to trace. First, the vast majority of medical services are still paid for on a fee-for-service basis. This system gives doctors incentives to perform

[7]Since neoconservative theorists generally ignore the contribution of the "medical and industrial complex"—i.e., the giant pharmaceutical companies, manufacturers of biomedical technology, hospital supply companies, etc.—to costs and inflation, their predictions of cost-containment through consumer choice appear rather unrealistic. A recent study by Harold Luft indicates that reliance on an HMO strategy will not affect the *rate* of escalation in health care costs. See Luft, "Trends in Medical Care Costs: Do HMOs Lower the Rate of Growth?" *Medical Care*, XIX (January 1980), 1–16.

[8]The conservative critique of medical market failure echoes some familiar themes in radical and mainstream liberal accounts. See, from left to center, Louise Lander, *National Health Insurance: A Health/PAC Report* (New York: Health Policy Advisory Center, 1975); Paul Starr and Gosta Esping-Andersen, "Passive Intervention,"*Working Papers*, July–August, 1979, pp. 15–25; and Karen Davis, *National Health Insurance* (Washington, D.C.: The Brookings Institution, 1975).

as many services as possible for as many patients as possible with little or no regard for cost. The second major problem stems from a concession to hospital interests. Under both Blue Cross and Medicare, payments to hospitals are based on reported costs. The more a particular hospital spends, the more it receives; therefore hospitals have no incentives to cut costs. Finally, and perhaps most important, the cost of the vast majority of medical transactions is borne not by the principals involved but by third parties. Since insurance companies pick up the medical tab, no one else in the system—patients, doctors, hospitals—has to reckon with the true costs of care; therefore no one has an incentive to save. Although they admit the importance of other factors such as general inflation and enormously expensive new medical technologies, Enthoven and others point to this complex of "perverse incentives" as the main cause of skyrocketing medical costs.

The present market is not only inflationary but also grossly inequitable. Professor Clark Havighurst, a leading health policy theorist, argues that the ultimate cause of our system's failure is the government's abdication of its wealth redistribution function in favor of the medical profession and private charity.[9] Enthoven is likewise critical of the many sources of inequity in the present system.[10] (References to Enthoven's *Health Plan* will be indicated by page numbers in parentheses in the text.) No one denies that there are pronounced disparities between the care received by people in urban and rural areas, between the urban middle class and the inner city, and even between the poor of different states. In spite of massive amounts of public monies earmarked for health

[9]Clark C. Havighurst, "Health Maintenance Organizations and the Market for Health Services," *Law and Contemporary Problems*, XXXV (1971), 741.

[10]Alain Enthoven, *Health Plan: The Only Practical Solution to the Soaring Cost of Medical Care* (Reading, Mass.: Addison-Wesley, 1980), pp. xvi, 117–18, and 139. Given the overwhelming complexity of the problems of rising costs, inflation, and inequity, this subtitle conveys unbridled hubris!

care, large gaps in coverage persist. As of 1975, over 6 million people below the poverty line were ineligible for Medicaid,[11] and in 1978, nearly 8% of the American population had no health insurance at all. Since our system relies so heavily on employer contributions to employees' health insurance, the holders of high-paying jobs and members of industrial unions receive more comprehensive and more expensive insurance than lower-paid workers in marginal nonunionized industries. Most workers who are laid off cannot afford to retain private health insurance; when they lose their jobs, they lose their coverage.

Enthoven's analysis of our irrational financing systems and inequitable distribution of health care reinforces the widely shared belief that the status quo is untenable. He suggests two broad strategies of reform: we can, he says, either press on with more government regulation—which could easily culminate in socialized medicine—or we can rely on market competition and reformed incentives. The latter is, of course, his preferred solution. (Enthoven does not even consider a third option—socialized medicine.)

The Free-Market Health Strategy

Based on their critique of the current delivery system, the primary objectives of the new proposals are twofold: (1) to reduce the costs of medical care through a system of rational economics and (2) to achieve a meaningful standard of equity in the delivery of health services.

Cost Containment through Rational Economics

Enthoven and Havighurst suggest that our present system must be replaced by a free market consisting mainly of competing

[11]Davis, *National Health Insurance*, p. 2; Enthoven, *Health Plan*, p. xvi.

organized health systems. These organizations would accept responsibility for providing comprehensive health care to a defined population, usually in return for prospective per capita payments. Although they are quite willing to include any worthwhile variations on this basic theme, Enthoven and Havighurst cite the Health Maintenance Organization (HMO) as the paradigmatic example of a cost-effective health care system.[12] But whatever the actual details, the new modes of delivery must provide incentives for everyone to economize.

The government's role is to facilitate a public solution to the health care crisis through the manipulation of private incentives. A central tenet of the new health policy is that government should get out of the business of providing or regulating services. Instead, it should limit itself to encouraging private providers to organize efficiently so as to attract cost-conscious consumers. The obvious vehicle for changing these private incentives is the tax system.

Enthoven proposes that we replace the present inequitable tax system—which excludes employer contributions from employees' taxable incomes—with a uniform system of refundable tax credits. Under such a scheme, the nonpoor would pay for their health care package with after-tax dollars, but they would receive a tax credit equal to 60% of the family's actuarial cost to help offset the expense.[13] Tax credits could be claimed only by members of government-approved health plans.

Because the credit would cover only 60% of actuarial costs,

[12]For two useful reviews of the concept, present standing, and prospects of HMOs, see Ernest W. Saward and Scott Fleming, "Health Maintenance Organizations," *Scientific American*, CCXLIII (October 1980), 47–53; and Harold S. Luft, "Assessing the Evidence on HMO Performance," *Milbank Memorial Fund Quarterly*, LVIII (Fall, 1980), 501–36.

[13]As defined by Enthoven, *actuarial cost* is the "average per capita cost for covered services for persons in each actuarial category." An "actuarial category" is a set of people—distinguished by age, sex, geographical location, etc.—for purposes of premium rating (Enthoven, *Health Plan*, pp. 119–20).

individuals would have a strong incentive to buy into less expensive plans, such as HMOs. Consumers could purchase more
expensive policies if they desired, but they would have to pay
the difference out of their own pockets. Thus, Enthoven expects
such cost-saving arrangements to eclipse fee-for-service medicine
if given the chance to compete in a robust free market.[14]

Equity through Vouchers

Whereas old-line AMA conservatives devoted themselves to
rear-guard actions against group practice and NHI, the new conservatives see no contradiction between a free-market strategy
and NHI. In fact, they tend to link the moral legitimacy of a
market solution to the prior establishment of a fully funded health
plan for the poor.[15] Consequently, Enthoven's Consumer Choice
Health Plan features a voucher plan for those who cannot afford
to purchase insurance or membership in a qualified health plan.
Taken together, the tax credits and voucher plan would yield
something like a system of NHI within a free-market context.[16]

Enthoven's voucher plan would replace Medicaid but still
be administered by a federal welfare agency. Vouchers could only
be exchanged for premiums on qualified health plans that met
minimum federal requirements; their value would be related to
family income. For families with no income apart from welfare,

---

[14]See also Clark Havighurst, "Speculations on the Market's Future in Health
Care," *Regulating Health Facilities Construction*, edited by Clark Havighurst
(Washington, D.C.: American Enterprise Institute, 1974).

[15]Ibid., p. 249.

[16]Enthoven writes, "The issue is not whether or not to enact national health
isurance (NHI). This country already has a sort of NHI system, with separate
programs for such groups as the aged, poor, employed middle-class, veterans,
military and dependents. The issue today is 'what kind of NHI?' " "Consumer
Choice Health Plan," *New England Journal of Medicine*, CCXC (March 23,
1978), 653.

the voucher would cover 100% of actuarial cost; as a family's income gradually increased, the value of its health care voucher would decline accordingly. Under CCHP, vouchers would thus cover the cost of health care for the poor while still maintaining work incentives.

As a result of the cost-containment strategy of CCHP, the poor would be encouraged to spend their health care dollars frugally. Toward this end, both Enthoven and Havighurst agree that the poor should be allowed to benefit from cost-conscious behavior. If the value of a family's voucher exceeds the cost of its qualified health plan, the family should derive some sort of profit from the difference. They disagree, however, on the kind of benefit the family might derive from its frugality. Havighurst favors a system of cash rebates that would allow families to pocket the difference between their vouchers and their health care premiums.[17] By contrast, Enthoven would either apply the surplus to more in-kind benefits (such as dental services) or leave the extra cash on deposit to offset future cost sharing (p. 123). This is a significant policy disagreement, and I shall return to it later.

Enthoven and Havighurst argue convincingly that such a combination of tax credits and vouchers would reallocate money from the rich to the poor much more directly and fairly than our present system. They point out, for example, that Medicare currently pays more money to the rich, who order more expensive care from more expensive health plans, than it does for the poor. They also contend, less convincingly, that the voucher plan will circumvent one of the more persistent and serious shortcomings of welfare medicine—the maintenance of a two-class system of care. Enthoven claims that vouchers—in combination with open enrollment in HMOs—will allow the poor to buy their way into

[17]Clark Havighurst, "Health Care Cost-Containment Regulation: Prospects and an Alternative," *American Journal of Law and Medicine*, II (1977), 321.

the "mainstream" of middle-class medicine. He has been somewhat evasive, however, concerning the precise level of equity
that we can expect from his voucher plan: CCHP would be a
"large step forward," he claims, even if it fell short of "a hypothetical egalitarian ideal" (p. 140).

In order to ensure an acceptable level of care in HMOs
serving those who pay through government vouchers, Havighurst
suggests that each HMO must enroll some minimum percentage
of private paying customers. This device, known as "proxy shopping," would thus require all HMOs to attract a substantial number of relatively sophisticated middle-class members before they
could treat patients with vouchers. In order to assure a decent
level of care for voucher recipients, Havighurst recommends that
qualified HMOs should enroll no less than 50% regular paying
customers.[18]

Defining Equity

Both Enthoven and Havighurst criticize the present system
for its inequities and adopt equity as a major design principle of
their health plans. What does equity mean and how likely is it
to be achieved through this new health care strategy? If the
standard of equity embodied in Enthoven's CCHP does not pretend to measure up to "a hypothetical egalitarian ideal," then
how far *does* it extend? In spite of their professed concern for
achieving equity, the new theorists manifest a surprising indifference to the problem of gauging, if only roughly, the content
of one or their guiding ideals. Typically, the term *equity* does
not even appear in the index of Enthoven's *Health Plan*.

This concept of equity has two separate dimensions: one
concerns the fair allocation of public funds among various eco-

nomic groups in society, while the other attempts to determine each individual's "fair share" of health benefits. When Enthoven charges that the present health care system is "inequitable," he usually has in mind the system of tax laws that subsidizes the purchase of health insurance—laws that generally favor the "well-insured well-to-do" rather than the working poor. As he rightly points out, a well-placed worker with a handsome package of health benefits may profit from a tax subsidy worth more than $1,000 a year, while a marginal worker in a marginal job gets no health benefits at all, and no subsidy (pp. 117–118).[19]

Enthoven concludes that we need a more equitable distribution of public funds. To achieve this goal, he advocates the establishment of a system of *uniform* tax credits that would bestow the same tax subsidy on the rich and (nearly) poor alike without regard for income or job status. (The size of the subsidy afforded the poor through vouchers would, of course, depend on family income.)

This proposed reform would clearly be an improvement over the status quo. It would route more money directly to the poor as a class and—by severing the connection between job and health insurance—it would help guarantee greater continuity of care for millions of Americans. But what does all this mean to the individual who happens to be poor and sick? Unless he or she is entitled to sufficient health care benefits, it will be small comfort to learn that the poor, as a group, will receive a fairer share of the wealth. What, then, does equity mean to the individual patient?

Although Enthoven and other market theorists provide an extremely vague concept of individual entitlement, they clearly and emphatically deny that equity should mean equality of access

[19]For a thorough treatment of the inequities inherent in most systems of tax incentives, see Stanley S. Surrey, "Tax Incentives as a Device for Implementing Government Policy: A Comparison with Direct Government Expenditures," *Harvard Law Review*, LXXXIII (February, 1970), 720–25.

or equal treatment. Since our society tolerates all sorts of significant inequalities—in education, housing, legal services, and
income—why, they ask, should we suddenly insist on equal treatment in health care?[20] That would be like asking why shouldn't
the poor have equal access to caviar at the Waldorf instead of
muddling by on food stamps? Still, this firm rejection of egalitarianism does not go so far as to commit the market theorists to
anything like a pure market solution, or, what comes to the same
thing, to an exclusive reliance on private charity to meet the
needs of the poor. Instead, their standard of equity for individuals
nestles vaguely between these extremes of egalitarianism and
laissez-faire liberalism. Following Charles Fried, we shall call
this the "decent minimum" standard.[21]

According to Fried, individuals should be free to purchase
whatever amount of health care they desire on the free market.
From this perspective, it would make no sense to say that we
spend too much or too little on health care; the right amount of
total spending for health care—on both the national and individual levels—would simply depend on how much we *desired* to
spend.[22] The poor would then be entitled to a decent minimum
through the voucher system. As sketched by Fried, "The decent
minimum should reflect some conception of what constitutes tolerable life prospects in general. It should speak quite strongly to
things like maternal and child health, which set the terms under
which individuals will compete and develop."[23] But what counts
as a decent minimum? What is the measure of tolerable life
prospects? And tolerable to whom—to Charles Fried of the Har-

[20]Charles Fried, "Equality and Rights in Medical Care," *Hastings Center Report*,
VI (February, 1976), 29–34. See also Alex Gerber, "Let's *Forget* About Equality
of Care," *Prism* III (October, 1975), 20–27.

[21]Ibid., p. 32.

[22]Charles Fried, "Health Care, Cost Containment, and Liberty" (paper delivered
at Hastings Center Conference On Ethics and Health Cost Containment, Washington, D.C., Oct. 3–5, 1978).

[23]Fried, "Equality and Rights," p. 32.

vard Law School, or to inner-city blacks whose life prospects are *already* intolerable?

While Enthoven is equally loath to address head-on the meaning of *minimal decency* in the medical context, he does provide, albeit indirectly, more of an answer than Fried. Since Enthoven's professed goal is to make middle-class, mainstream health care available to the poor through his voucher plan, his basic requirements for all qualified health plans—including the mandatory offering of a low option of basic health services—would seem to specify in a roundabout and hesitant way the list of minimal services implied by his notion of equity. Thus, he suggests that:

> A qualified health plan would be required to cover, at a minimum, the list of services called "basic health services" in the HMO Act of 1973 (as amended). That list includes physician services, inpatient and outpatient hospital services, emergency health services, short-term outpatient mental health services (up to twenty visits), treatment and referral for drug and alcohol abuse, laboratory, and X-ray, home health services, and certain preventive health services. (p. 128)

Although this list was originally formulated with middle-class consumers in mind, it would also presumably function as a standard of minimally decent care for the poor under CCHP. Enthoven is quick to add, however, that there is nothing sacred about this particular set of services and that a less costly list might well make sense. Thus, his notion of minimal decency, while more explicit than Fried's, is still quite vague and subject to political bargaining.

The Rawlsian Perspective

This standard of equity is attractive to market theorists because it fosters freedom of choice while still responding to a sense of responsibility for meeting the most desperate needs of the poor. In order to situate this conception of equity within the current intellectual landscape, it might be helpful to compare it briefly with the most noticeable landmark—John Rawls's theory of distributive justice.[24]

According to Rawls, significant social and economic inequalities are permissible, but only if they are both (1) reasonably expected to be to everyone's advantage, including those who are least well off, and (2) attached to positions and offices open to all. While Rawls's "difference principle" does not demand strict equality, it justifies only those inequalities that improve the position of all concerned. If the basic structure of our economy rewards the wealthy with an unequal distribution that does not eventually redound to the benefit of the worst off, or (worse still) if the "haves" directly benefit at the expense of the "have nots," then our society falls short of Rawlsian justice. Likewise, if certain basic needs—including health care needs—go unfulfilled, then equality of opportunity becomes an empty formality, and those who enter society with a competitive disadvantage only become increasingly disadvantaged. Rawlsian justice appears to require that all such basic needs be met in a relatively affluent society.[25]

On some points, the neoconservatives and Rawls do not seem so far apart. While they have little use for Rawls's difference principle or for his notion of fair equality of opportunity, the market theorists approach a Rawlsian attitude when they concentrate on the interests of the least well off while tolerating rather large differences between social classes. In addition, al-

[24]John Rawls, A Theory of Justice (Cambridge, Mass.: Harvard University Press, 1971), p. 60.

[25]I have drawn here from my previous discussion of Rawlsian justice and health care in "Ethical Theory in the Medical Context" Ethical Issues in Modern Medicine, edited by John Arras and Robert Hunt (2nd ed.; Palo Alto, Calif.: Mayfield, 1983), pp. 19–22. See also Norman Daniels, "Health-Care Needs and Distributive Justice," Philosophy and Public Affairs, X (Spring, 1981), 146–79.

though Rawls is more concerned to hitch the fortunes of the rich to the prospects of the poor—thereby delimiting the former's freedom of choice—some of his statements on the background institutions required by justice seem to invite Fried's "minimalist" formula. Rawls states, for example, that the government should guarantee a social minimum through special payments for sickness and other income subsidies.[26]

While I cannot give a lengthy analysis of competing theories of justice, I want to point out some deficiencies in this "minimal decency" standard when seen from a more egalitarian vantage point. As its name implies, a theory that mandates minimally decent shares must necessarily allow for (at least) a two-class system of medical care. Despite all the rhetoric depicting the poor floating down the medical mainstream atop their vouchers, the neoconservatives are obviously committed to a stratified system of health care. Whether such inequality amounts to inequity depends upon one's larger theory of distributive justice.

For Rawlsians, the degree of inequality contemplated by the minimal decency standard would clearly be inequitable. Although Fried's standard does focus attention on Rawls's "least advantaged" class, it effectively severs the moral and economic bonds linking the "have nots" with the "haves"—a bond forged by Rawls's difference principle. Whereas Rawls insists that any inequalities enjoyed by the rich should also benefit the poor, Fried's theory will tolerate any and all inequalities as long as the basic needs of the poor have been met. In this respect, Fried's theory bears a closer resemblance to the libertarianism of Robert Nozick than it does to Rawls's views.[27]

An even more serious criticism of Fried's standard can be launched from Rawls's requirement of equal opportunity. Rawls

[26]Rawls, A Theory of Justice, p. 275.
[27]Robert Nozick, Anarchy, State and Utopia (New York: Basic Books, 1974).

is not content with a merely "formal" equality of opportunity—
that is, with systems that allow people to exploit fully for their
own personal benefit not only their (unearned) natural talents
but also all the (unfair) advantages that accrue from membership
in a privileged social class. He opts for a system of "fair" equality
of opportunity, which attempts to mitigate (as far as possible) the
effects of such natural and social competitive advantages.[28] Thus,
even though Rawls is quite willing to allow the market to determine each person's final allotment of goods, he insists that institutions guaranteeing genuinely fair competition be established
beforehand.

Judged against this notion of equal opportunity, Fried's concept of minimal decency seems clearly deficient and inequitable.
Despite the vagueness of Fried's notion of "tolerable life prospects in general," such a standard clearly would allow unearned
natural and social advantages to play a large role in the allocation
of desirable roles in society; it would also effectively reinforce
existing class barriers that make it especially difficult for the poor
to compete in the free market. Moreover, with regard to the
distribution of health care, Fried's standard would not only dis-
criminate unfairly against poor and elderly victims of chronic
illness but also set a standard of care well below requirements
of genuinely equal opportunity for the youthful poor. One could,
I suppose, live a "tolerable life in general" from a wheelchair.[29]

Other political theories are even more egalitarian than Rawls's.
Robert Veatch's theory of medical justice, for example, condemns
all two-class systems—including those that would satisfy the difference principle—on the ground that they allow basic inequal-

[28]Rawls, A Theory of Justice, pp. 72–75.
[29]Fried's views on social justice in health care have changed rather dramatically
in the last decade. In an earlier book, Medical Experimentation (New York:
Elsevier, 1974), Fried eloquently argued for a full-fledged right to health care
on the basis of a prior right to genuine equality of opportunity!

ities which are unjustifiable among equals. From this perspective, the two-class system espoused by the neoconservatives would be unjust even if it provided substantial benefits for the poor.[30]

What are the prospects of achieving equity (as defined by Fried and Enthoven) through the NHI–voucher strategy? I shall argue that this strategy offers little or nothing to precisely those social groups whose welfare often serves as an index of equity and social justice—the medically underserved rural populations and the urban poor.

The Health Care Market in Rural America

In 1976 over 53 million Americans lived in roughly 900 rural counties, which together comprise about 40% of the land mass of this country. These areas are characterized by low population density, a disproportionate share of the country's poor and elderly, and shortages of all kinds. Most important for our purposes, however, are the critical shortages of health manpower and health services delivery systems.

In 1977 rural areas averaged less than one primary care physician for every 3,500 people.[31] According to one source, the number of physicians in rural areas decreased from 1967 to 1977, while the number of counties without functional access to primary care increased by nearly 35% between 1970 and 1977. While rural America was facing this decline in available medical ser-

---

[30]Personal communication from Robert Veatch. See also "What Is a 'Just' Health Care Delivery?" *Ethics And Health Policy*, edited by Robert Veatch and Roy Branson (Cambridge, Mass.: Ballinger, 1976), pp. 127–53.

[31]Edward Martin, M.D., "Consumer Choice Health Plan: Impact on Rural America," *Effects of the Payment Mechanism on the Health Care Delivery System* edited by William R. Roy, DHEW Publication No. (PHS) 78-3227 (Washington, D.C.: U.S. Department of Health, Education, and Welfare, 1978), pp. 47–48.

vices, the total number of practicing physicians in the United States actually increased by 14%!

Although Enthoven bemoans the inequitable geographical distribution that leaves most rural populations poorly served,[32] his health plan does not attempt a direct solution. True to his faith in the private sector, he only expresses a vague hope that more and more doctors will settle in rural areas in response to market pressures generated by CCHP in urban areas. Competition is expected to narrow the range of acceptable opportunities in the cities and eventually squeeze many of the surplus physicians out into rural practices.[33]

Presumably, additional motivation for this medical migration will come from the system of tax credits and vouchers, which will give rural residents the purchasing power they need to outfit their new physicians in Ralph Lauren boots, chaps, and Land Rovers. Unfortunately, the only empirical evidence Enthoven adduces in defense of this speculative scenario is drawn from the experience of Kaiser-Permanente, which operates remote outposts in the Hawaiian Islands (p. 140).

While Enthoven is certainly entitled to his speculations, others—who have relegated the "invisible hand" to the company of the Tooth Fairy and other mythical beasts—have good reason to be less sanguine about CCHP bringing equity to rural America. Until we know more about the real forces and motivations underlying physicians' choice of location, we can do little more than speculate about the future. Still we must be careful to distinguish faith from experience and historical probabilities.

Consider first the sparseness of most rural populations—a factor that will most likely discourage investors and impede the development of competition among health plans. Contrary to the

[32]Enthoven, "Consumer Choice Health Plan," p. 65.
[33]See Walter McClure's comments on this theme in Roy, ed., *Effects of the Payment Mechanism*, p. 57.

theory of CCHP, huge expanses of rural America would become strictly a seller's market, thus defeating the cost-cutting goals of the program.

Even more disturbing, however, is the prospect that in many rural areas no health services at all would be offered.[34] The lack of physicians' services will most likely undercut any market-oriented solution to the problem of rural underservice. Will an anticipated glut of physicians in urban areas lead to the expected migration of doctors to the country? The research findings on this question are mixed and inconclusive. Most policy analysts deny that the medical care market resembles other markets. They suggest that an oversupply of physicians in desirable areas will merely produce more specialization, thereby encouraging doctors to work less, charge more, and require more stimulating work environments.[35] This pattern will most likely be abetted by our system of medical education, which discourages general family practice in favor of specialized, highly technological, and hospital-based medicine. As for Enthoven's one example of rural outreach by Kaiser, Edward Martin cogently points out: "We've got to go back to the heterogeneity of rural America. I mean, going to Maui is not exactly the same as going to Rotten Creek, Montana."[36] According to this view, as long as we depend on the good will of physicians reinforced by weak and indirect market incentives, we cannot reasonably expect a medical exodus.

This standard theory of medical manpower distribution has

[34]James D. Bernstein, "Comment" in Roy, *Effects of the Payment Mechanism*, p. 53. See also Luft, "Assessing the Evidence on HMO Performance," pp. 521–24.

[35]See, for example, John P. Bunker, "Surgical Manpower: A Comparison of Operations and Surgeons in the United States and in England and Wales," *New England Journal of Medicine*, CCLXXIII (1970), 135 ff.; and U. E. Reinhardt, *Physician Productivity and the Demand for Health Services: An Economic Analysis* (Cambridge, Mass.: Ballinger, 1975).

[36]Martin, "Consumer Choice Health Plan," p. 58.

not gone uncontested. In a recently published Rand Corporation study, William B. Schwartz and his colleagues challenge the conventional wisdom, echoed above, that market pressures will not force doctors to practice in rural areas.[37] These authors have amassed large amounts of data suggesting that the board-certified physicians *are* diffusing into nonmetropolitan areas and that market forces provide the best explanation of this phenomenon. The Rand study thus challenges two fundamental assumptions undergirding current health manpower policies: (1) the belief that physicians can effectively create a demand for their services, thereby shielding themselves from the effects of competition, and (2) the view that physicians can avoid the necessity of migrating to rural areas through the temporizing strategy of specialization. Schwartz's data purportedly show that doctors are not immune to competition and that specialization retards, but does not prevent, diffusion of doctors into rural areas. Consequently, he predicts substantial further diffusion of physicians from 1977 to 1985. The likelihood of this occurring is enhanced by two factors: (1) the number of physicians will increase by 30% during this period and (2) the likely adoption of some form of NHI will provide rural populations with attractive purchasing power. A script worthy of Alain Enthoven!

Others may criticize Schwartz's claims on demographic and economic grounds, but even if we grant the central points of the Rand study, two problems remain. First, as Schwartz himself admits, we still do not know how the diffusion patterns described in this study affect the rural population's access to care. Are physicians diffusing to the *right places* and at a *satisfactory rate* to rectify present inequities in a reasonable period of time? Second, there is a problem concerning the efficient investment of

[37]William B. Schwartz, Joseph P. Newhouse, Bruce W. Bennett, and Albert P. Williams, "The Changing Geographic Distribution of Board-Certified Physicians," *New England Journal of Medicine* CCXCII (Oct. 30, 1980), 1032–38.

public monies in health manpower training. Schwartz's data seem to indicate that if we keep increasing the number of medical college graduates each year, a sufficient number will eventually be squeezed out of the metropolitan market in spite of their best efforts to stay (for example, through specialization). If Schwartz's predictions are accurate, the rural health manpower shortage *could* be rectified—but at what cost? How many new physicians must we train at great expense in order to coax the requisite number out of the city and into the country? At what point would this indirect, market-oriented strategy become excessively expensive and irrational from a policy perspective?

Rural areas also lack health service delivery systems. Vouchers might well provide rural residents with ample purchasing power, but there will most likely be nothing for them to purchase in the absence of established health systems. As Theodore Marmor observes, "Other Western democracies have learned that poor distribution remains even after the medical purchasing power of . . . rural areas [is] improved."[38] The barriers to health care have remained largely intact in those countries—such as Canada, Germany, and Finland—that have emphasized financing while ignoring the development of health delivery systems. By contrast, countries that have addressed both the financial and functional obstacles to health care—such as Denmark—have succeeded in achieving greater equity.[39] In view of these international lessons, Enthoven's unwillingness to contemplate government grants and subsidies for health systems development seems to be ultimately self-defeating (p. 134). If we are serious about remedying medical underservice in rural areas—many of whose residents fit Rawls's category of the "least advantaged"—then we should adopt a strategy of direct action, either by providing incentives that *will* attract

[38]Theodore Marmor, "Rethinking National Health Insurance," *The Public Interest*, Winter, 1977, pp. 83–84.
[39]Martin, "Consumer Choice Health Plan," p. 49.

needed personnel and health systems or by direct governmental provision of services.[40]

The Health Needs of the Urban Poor

Although neither Enthoven nor Havighurst[41] is strongly optimistic about a market solution to rural health care needs, both assert that the NHI–voucher strategy will provide an equitable solution to the problems of welfare medicine in the inner cities. One extremely problematical assumption behind such optimism is a belief in consumer sovereignty, not merely among the middle class (itself a debatable point) but also among the urban poor. Can we assume that the poor will satisfy their genuine health needs in a voucher system, even as they respond to the cost-saving incentives of CCHP? Or is there embedded in the very structure of CCHP a fundamental contradiction between the goals of rational economics and equity?

Enthoven and Havighurst might well be startled by such questions, since they never explicitly raise the issue of meeting health *needs*. CCHP and its kin are delivery systems designed to satisfy wants, not needs.[42] While a system geared to alleviating medical needs would concentrate on significant physical or psychological malfunctions—most likely giving substantial authority to experts trained to detect them—a system geared to satisfying wants would try to give patient–consumers whatever they hap-

[40]Robert Lekachman defends this preference for direct action against relying on long chains of causal sequences in his essay "Economic Justice in Hard Times," *Ethics in Hard Times,* edited by Arthur Caplan and Daniel Callahan (New York: Plenum Press, 1981).

[41]Havighurst concedes that rural areas would require special public investment beyond vouchers. "HMOs and the Market for Health Services," pp. 752–53.

[42]For a careful discussion of this distinction between "needs" and "wants" in health care, see Daniels, "Health-Care Needs and Distributive Justice."

pened to desire (providing they could pay for it), from neuro-surgery to nose jobs. There is nothing particularly disturbing about this emphasis on wants as long as people *want* to satisfy their *needs*—or if they do not, as long as their choices are genuinely free and uncoerced. The problem for Enthoven and Havighurst is that *neither* of these two conditions would exist for the urban poor under CCHP.

Consider the following sketch of the urban poor. First, the poor experience more illness and have greater health needs than do the members of the middle and upper classes. A wealth of statistical surveys indicates, for example, that the infant mortality rate of poverty areas is 50% higher than that of nonpoverty areas; that tuberculosis is three times more prevalent in poverty areas; that young adults and middle-aged people earning less than $5,000 per year had 30% more chronic illness and 50% higher rates of diabetes, hypertension, and visual impairment than people in the same age cohort earning more than $15,000; and that disability is strongly correlated with poverty.[43]

Second, serious doubts can be raised about the ability of the urban poor to make fully informed decisions regarding health care in a context of economic deprivation. If relatively affluent suburbanites have trouble negotiating their way through a market characterized by consumer uncertainty and ignorance of quality,[44] then we should expect the urban poor to fare even worse. Lack of knowledge regarding the predictability of disease and the quality of medical services is a serious impediment to consumer

[43]Some of these studies are discussed in David A. Kindig, Victor W. Sidel, and Irwin Birnbaum, "National Health Insurance for Inner City Underserved Areas: General Criteria and Analysis of a Proposed Administrative Mechanism," in Roy, ed., *Effects of the Payment Mechanism*, pp. 60–66. See also M. H. Rudov and Nancy Santangelo's report to DHEW, *Health Status of Minorities and Low-Income Groups* (Washington: U.S. Government Printing Office, 1979).

[44]Kenneth Arrow, "Uncertainty and the Welfare Economics of Medical Care," *The American Economic Review*, LIII (December, 1963), 948–54.

sovereignty, and thus to a market solution, among rich and poor alike.

Third, whereas ignorance concerning medical services cuts across class boundaries—albeit more or less deeply—medical sociologists and other critics have found that health priorities (that is, the attitudes of people toward their own health) are directly and strongly related to social class.[45] Those with sufficient incomes to cover their basic physical needs will generally insist on freedom from pain and discomfort and are likely to be interested in maintaining their health through preventive measures. The poor, by contrast, must cope with a minimum of physical necessities; when given an option, they tend to prefer such things as better living conditions and improved transportation to more health care. According to this sociological literature, the poor tend to equate "health" with the ability to keep on working. Thus preventive care and treatment for minor illnesses do not ordinarily figure in the health care picture of the urban poor. Economic deprivation thus renders the poor unable to appreciate either their own health needs or the potential benefits of medical care. As Richard Lichtman, a Marxist social critic, puts it, "Our economic system so maldistributes wealth that men are radically unequal in their capacity to provide for their own health and unevenly positioned even to grasp its significance."[46]

Fourth, welfare recipients differ markedly from the middle class in their ability to surmount bureaucratic obstacles and effect institutional change. Large, impersonal welfare agencies generally tend to foster passive behavior on the part of their clients.

[45]For a helpful overview of the literature on this question, see *The Health Gap: Medical Services and the Poor*, edited by Robert Kane, Josephine Kasteler, and Robert Gray (New York: Springer, 1976), pp. 3–21.

[46]Richard Lichtman, "The Political Economy of Medical Care," *The Social Organization of Health*, edited by Hans Peter Dreitzel (New York: Macmillan, 1971), p. 267.

Compared to members of the middle class—many of whom are bureaucrats themselves, familiar with the levers of power—the average welfare recipient is just not experienced in registering complaints and forcing institutions to be more responsive to his or her needs.

These sociological observations should not be construed as attempts to "blame the victim." The poor have no choice about paying for food, clothing, and rent, but they *can* postpone medical services. Thus, we need not assume that the poor do not know what they are doing or do not value medicine; we need merely recognize that some expenses can be put off while others cannot. The low priority the poor allot to health care is not necessarily an indicator of how they actually *value* medicine or of how they *define* disease; rather, it reflects urgency born of economic coercion.

This sketch of the urban poor suggests that there is a rather wide gap separating the rhetoric of consumer sovereignty from the realities of inner-city life. The HMO strategy depends for its success on a clientele that is (1) relatively well informed, (2) appreciative of the value of medical services, (3) sufficiently affluent to place health services on a par with other basic necessities, and (4) sufficiently assertive to ensure institutional responsiveness to consumer preferences. But inner-city HMOs can be expected to enroll a clientele that is relatively uneducated about health care; that either undervalues medical services or is too poor to rank them on a par with food, shelter, and rent; and that is generally docile in the face of institutional ineptitude and neglect. What sort of behavior can we expect from such consumers in the context of a health care system that has, until quite recently, exclusively served middle-class populations?

Let us first assume the implementation of an HMO program that features Havighurst's cash rebate. Given such an arrangement, we should expect the urban poor to buy into the cheapest possible health care plans. If the poor generally assign lower priority to health care than to the provision of food, clothing, and shelter, and if they can expect a cash rebate from the purchase of less expensive (and therefore less comprehensive) health care plans, then it would be rational for the poor to buy the cheapest, least comprehensive package they can find. Thus, those in the greatest medical need will be compelled by a combination of economic adversity and monetary incentives to buy into health plans whose options will fail to meet their greater-than-average health care needs.

Enthoven's remedy for the predictable failure of a cash rebate plan is to reward cost-conscious welfare consumers with more in-kind services—such as dentistry, eyeglasses, or drugs—in case their premiums fall short of the full value of their vouchers. In addition, Enthoven is prepared to set standards for qualified health care plans that would establish a minimum acceptable level of services for all consumers. Assuming that the level is set high enough to provide for everyone's basic health care needs, CCHP would insure a decent level of care for the poor while maintaining incentives for cost-saving behavior (pp. 138–140). Enthoven's proposed remedy does not, however, anticipate the likely scenario of the near poor choosing not to supplement their vouchers with their own money. Given oppressive economic circumstances, many near-poor people might not be able to afford to supplement partial vouchers worth some fraction of a policy's full cost. Their vouchers would, in effect, be wasted, and they would not be insured against ill health.

The Experience of Welfare Medicine

While this proposal represents a theoretical advance over Havighurst's self-defeating cash rebate scheme, it is nevertheless subject to more practical objections. The ability of CCHP to meet the health care needs of the urban poor would depend upon the level of its floor—that is, upon its conception of a "decent minimum" package of basic services that all qualified plans would have to provide. Would this floor be set high enough in practice under CCHP? The discouraging history of welfare medicine in this country suggests a negative answer.

Remember that CCHP's voucher plan would be administered by the federal welfare system (p. 123). Although our system of welfare medicine was theoretically supposed to provide greater equity for the poor, in practice welfare programs have constantly been eroded by cutbacks and the exclusion of the needy poor. As Robert and Rosemary Stevens amply demonstrate in their magisterial study, *Welfare Medicine in America,* cost containment and eligibility—rather than the meeting of health care needs— soon became the major policy questions determining the form and extent of welfare medicine in America.[47] The Stevenses not only show in depressing detail how the legitimate health-related goals of Medicare and Medicaid have been thwarted by budgetary concerns but also point out that, in practice, both programs came to be dominated by fiscal objectives. Medicare served to maintain the incomes of the deserving elderly that were threatened by high medical bills, while Medicaid served largely to help get the sick poor off the welfare rolls. The fate of welfare medicine was closely linked to fiscal, rather than humanitarian, objectives.

No wonder that public support of welfare medicine has fluctuated with the economic and political winds. Undoubtedly the policy analysts responsible for such programs (including CCHP) have been motivated primarily by humanitarian ideals; but the inner logic of welfare medicine, as exhibited in the history of Medicaid, has consistently confounded the best of intentions.

---

[47]Robert Stevens and Rosemary Stevens, *Welfare Medicine in America: A Case Study of Medicaid* (New York: The Free Press, 1974), p. 53.

The lesson here is that CCHP will probably not succeed in establishing a meaningful standard of basic health care in this country as long as it is placed under the rubric of welfare. In order to avoid this conclusion, Enthoven must explain how CCHP will correct the deficiencies of Medicaid in achieving equitable funding levels. Given the present state of our economy and the rising tide of antiwelfare opinion in this country, Enthoven bears a heavy burden of proof indeed.[48]

The Poor and Second-Class Medicine

At this point Professor Havighurst might object that my argument is a non sequitur. He might claim that, even if I am right about the poor lacking consumer sovereignty, equity can still be achieved through his plan. Recall that whereas Enthoven offered only vague predictions that the poor would end up with more than second-class care, Havighurst's plan attempts to provide mainstream care for the poor through the device of proxy shopping. Since this mechanism would require all HMOs to enroll at least 50% regular paying customers before they could accept welfare vouchers, Havighurst could argue that the poor do not need to be "sovereign customers"; they can simply rely on the regular paying customers to "work the system" for them. Even if the poor did not know the difference between high- and low-quality medicine, they could count on their "proxies" to insist on rigorous standards of expertise and surroundings that respected their dignity as human beings.

---

[48]This burden has been made heavier still by the recent proposals of Enthoven's advisee in the White House. President Reagan currently intends to slash $1.3 billion from former President Carter's original Medicaid request of $18.8 billion. Cf. *Congressional Quarterly Weekly Report*, Vol. 39, No. 16 (April 18, 1981).

But this argument, like the theory of consumer sovereignty, is out of touch with reality. In order for proxy shopping to achieve the desired effect, the recipients of welfare medicine would have to be more or less evenly distributed throughout the population. Yet welfare recipients tend to cluster in densely populated and run-down regions of large metropolitan areas. Since the urban middle class can reasonably be expected to continue frequenting its own neighborhood and suburban health facilities, where will the proxy shoppers for welfare HMOs be found? Will they, one wonders, be bused in from the suburbs? If proxy shoppers are not forthcoming, then inner-city HMOs will presumably fail to qualify for the federal voucher plan and the urban poor will find themselves in the same position as rural populations, equipped with vouchers that they cannot redeem.

Thus, Havighurst confronts the following dilemma: he can insist either on high-quality care for the poor through proxy shopping or on mere access to second-class care. If he opts for a quality system, the poor will not have access to medical care; if he opts to guarantee access (by dispensing with the proxy-shopping requirement), he must settle for a low-quality, second-class system. Given the geographical distribution of the poor and the unwillingness of the middle class to serve as proxies, Havighurst cannot have it both ways.

The recent performance of "Medicaid HMOs" (HMOs expressly established to serve Medicaid patients) in California lends support to this troubling conclusion. Apparently moved by the belief that switching to more cost-effective HMOs would save millions in welfare funds while minimizing the role of government, California legislators in 1971 passed the Medical Reform Act—a law that facilitated the rapid transfer of Medi-Cal recipients to prepaid health plans. Since proxy shopping was not required of these providers, mere access to care was no problem: as early as 1973, 55 HMOs had enrolled 237,000 Medi-Cal clients.

But, as one might well expect, the quality of care was decidedly not "mainstream." Bruce Spitz, formerly of the Urban Institute, reported that

> as the HMO activity peaked, a series of state and federal investigations revealed program irregularities. Inappropriate and fraudulent HMO marketing practices were common. . . . There were indications of gross under-utilization of services. . . . Horror stories abound about denials of emergency care and poor treatment.[49]

The care administered in these welfare HMOs was not merely poor, it was also much more expensive than had been anticipated. In fact, two of the largest health care contractors charged the state capitation rates that were as high or higher than ordinary fee-for-service rates in the same areas. A study of 15 such plans by the California Auditor General showed that, on the average, 52% of the state-funded capitation payments (a total of $56 million) went into administrative expenses and profits.[50] This compares poorly with the experience of other HMOs that spend roughly 10% of the premium dollar on administrative costs. While intensive regulation by the state might possibly curb such anomalous spending patterns, it would certainly be at odds with the antiregulative thrust of medical neoconservatism.

Predictably, Enthoven attributes the welfare HMO disaster in California to "the government's politically motivated purchasing policies," rather than to the nature of HMOs (pp. 68–69). He argues that it is unfair to view the California experience as representative of HMOs, just as it would be unfair to judge the quality of fee-for-service medicine on the basis of the equally scandalous "Medicaid mills."

---

[49]Bruce Spitz, "When a Solution is Not a Solution: Medicaid and Health Maintenance Organizations," *Journal of Health Politics, Policy and Law*, III (Winter, 1979), 512–13.

[50]Charles Lewis reports this study in "Health-Maintenance Organizations: Guarantors of Access to Medical Care?" in *A Right to Health: The Problem of Access to Primary Care*, edited by Charles Lewis, Rashi Fein, and David Mechanic (New York: Wiley–Interscience, 1976), p. 236.

Of course, Enthoven is right; it *would* be unfair to generalize from a welfare HMO scandal to the conclusion that *all* HMOs are necessarily expensive and underserve their patients. On the contrary, we should *expect* a system designed for the middle class to function irregularly in poverty areas. But this is precisely the problem which Enthoven's response completely ignores. In order to assess the impact of CCHP on the poor, we need to know how representative the California scandal is likely to be, not of HMOs *per se* but rather of HMOs in a context of welfare medicine. Even if advocates of the NHI–HMO strategy can successfully parry the standard general objections about probable HMO underservice,[51] they still have to grapple with the specific problems of underservice, low quality, and administrative fraud in Medicaid-type HMOs. Concerning these, Enthoven is silent, and the historical record is not reassuring.

Since its inception in 1965, Medicaid has done little to homogenize our two-class system of health care. Although the incidence of hard-core Medicaid mills may have been exaggerated, 60% of all Medicaid patients do receive their health care in large Medicaid practices (that is, those in which at least a third of the patients are on welfare) that are markedly inferior to mainstream care. According to a recent study by Janet Mitchell and Jerry Cromwell, the background and training of physicians engaged in welfare medicine differ substantially from those of other physicians: welfare physicians tend to be older, less specialized, less

---

[51] A commonplace charge against HMOs is that their system of financial incentives encourages underservice, just as fee-for-service encourages overservice. See *Prognosis Negative: Crisis in the Health Care System*, edited by David Kotelchuck (New York: Vintage, 1976), pp. 359–63. As a satisfied customer of HMOs in New York and Southern California, I have never been particularly impressed by this sweeping charge. Nevertheless, the more vulnerable an HMO's population, the more suspicious we should be that profits are being reaped through underservice. See Elliott Krause's (admittedly anecdotal) evidence to this effect in "Capitalism, Costs, and the Shape of Service: Reply to a Critique," *Journal of Health Politics, Policy and Law*, II (Winter, 1978), 588–90.

credentialed, and more often trained in foreign medical schools than their counterparts in the mainstream. And although the poor have greater health needs, they generally receive shorter visits and fewer ancillary health services (lab tests, injections, X-ray exams, and office surgery) than middle- and upper-class patients. Mitchell and Cromwell observe:

> the Medicaid program and its beneficiaries constitute a secondary, residual market, subordinate to the better-paying primary market. More highly trained physicians face greater demand for their services and are able to see private patients who are willing to pay higher fees. Competition for patients drives less-qualified physicians into the Medicaid program in disproportionate numbers. A primary goal of the Medicaid program—to integrate the poor into mainstream medicine—is thereby thwarted.[52]

Although Enthoven cites one example of an apparently successful prepaid plan for low-income people—Project Health of Multnomah County, Oregon (pp. 88–89)—he gives us no reason to think that a nationwide network of large Medicaid-type practices would overcome the entrenched two-tiered system described by Mitchell and Cromwell. Such large-scale inequity is not threatened by isolated counterinstances of well-funded social experiments.

Equity through Vouchers?

If the leaders of this "counterrevolution" in health policy desire to do more than cut costs, if they also want to move toward a more equitable health care system, they would be well advised to recall previous attempts to achieve equity in health care through

[52]Janet B. Mitchell and Jerry Cromwell, "Large Medicaid Practices and Medicaid Mills," *Journal of the American Medical Association*, CCXLIV (Nov. 28, 1980), 2437.

vouchers. There is a familiar ring to the current rhetoric about
bringing the poor into the mainstream of American medicine,
because exactly the same things were said on behalf of Medicaid
prior to its passage in 1965. The liberal proponents of that ill-
fated program wrote the script for the medical conservatives of
the 1970s and 1980s. The basic problem, it was alleged, was that
the poor are poor; they lack the means to escape from the network
of second-class medicine. If the poor could just be provided with
sufficient funds—say, through vouchers—they would be able to
enter the medical mainstream. Through a system of vouchers,
the poor would receive the same quality of care, from the same
sources, as the rich.[53] The old two-class system of medical care
would simply wither away as Medicaid recipients abandoned the
lower tier in favor of first-class medicine.

Needless to say, the promise of Medicaid was never fulfilled.
Although this program did extend the benefits of medical care
to significant numbers of poor people who would otherwise have
gone without, it failed miserably to make good on its rhetoric of
equity and quality medicine for the poor. That health policy
analysts could have lived through this failure only to emerge in
the 1970s reciting from the same script testifies, I think, to the
powerful appeal of the voucher idea for American health planners.

The theory of vouchers is extremely attractive in part because it somehow manages to combine in a single plan the cher-
ished values of both the political left and right. For the medical
left wing, the voucher strategy offers an approximation of "the
right to health care" for the poor. And as Enthoven points out,
in conjunction with a system of uniform tax credits, the voucher
plan could finally realize the elusive ideal of NHI (of sorts). For
those on the medical right, vouchers stand for freedom of choice
and the virtues of the market. Vouchers thus appear to offer the

[53]Stevens and Stevens, *Welfare Medicine in America*, p. xvi.

prospect of a right to health care without governmental provision of services and a free market that actually cares for the poor. It is no wonder that vouchers emerged in the 1970s as the golden mean between "totalitarian" socialism and a heartless capitalism: it is the perfect *liberal individualist* solution to the health care crisis.

A Right without Foundations

It is highly unlikely that equity, even as defined by Enthoven and Havighurst, can be achieved through a voucher plan. Rural residents can be given vouchers, but in the absence of direct governmental incentives or provision of services, they will have no place to cash them in. For the urban poor, vouchers will represent a ticket to purchase more second-class care in degrading and dehumanizing circumstances. The "right to health care" would thus appear to be a right without genuine economic foundations. Just as liberal capitalism espouses a system of *negative* political rights and liberties without an accompanying charter of economic rights,[54] so now the advocates of medical capitalism present us with the odd spectacle of a specific *positive* right— the right to health care—that also lacks an adequate economic and institutional base. In each case, these liberal rights can be reduced to mere formalities in a context of free-market capitalism and deep class divisions. The poor might have a political right to travel, for example, but if they lack economic standing, this right will be worth little to them. Likewise, under CCHP the poor will have a formal "right" to health services that either will not

---

[54]Marx criticizes the system of liberal political rights in "On the Jewish Question," reprinted in *Karl Marx: Selected Writings*, edited by David McLellan (Oxford, England: Oxford University Press, 1977), pp. 39–62.

exist (in rural areas) or will be of markedly inferior quality (in the cities). This "right to health care" turns out to be an empty entitlement. Until legislators and health planners begin to take seriously the health needs of our medically underserved—a group whose number approximates the entire population of Great Britain—we shall no doubt continue to reconcile free enterprise and social justice by means of rhetoric.[55] For those with ears to hear beneath this rhetoric of equity, the neoconservative message is clear: "The poor have inadequate health care? Then let them eat vouchers!"

ACKNOWLEDGMENTS

I am indebted to a number of colleagues for their constructive criticisms. Special thanks to Thomas Murray, Nancy Rhoden, Arthur Caplan, Robert Veatch, Ruth Macklin, Margaret Steinfels, Ronald Bayer, Norman Daniels, and Leith Mullings. Grudging thanks to Ernest Tai for introducing me to the wonderful world of government documents.

[55]See Max Skidmore, *Medicare and the American Rhetoric of Reconcilition* (Tuscaloosa, Ala.: University of Alabama Press, 1970).

6

Robert L. Dickman

Operationalizing Respect for Persons

A QUALITATIVE ASPECT OF THE RIGHT TO HEALTH CARE

Introduction

"The right to health care" has, as a slogan, enjoyed a great deal of popularity in this country as well as internationally for over a decade. In 1970, the World Health Assembly declared without qualification that "the right to health is a fundamental human right."[1] The slogan has also served (and continues to serve) as a basic rallying point for those eager to call for or to effect reform in our health care delivery system.[2] Thus, it remains as the initial jumping-off point for numerous comprehensive national health insurance proposals as well as a major tenet of activist community

[1]Victor Sidel, "The Right to Health Care: An International Perspective," *Bioethics and Human Rights*, edited by Elsie Bandman and Bertram Bandman (Boston: Little, Brown, 1978), p. 342.
[2]Ibid. p. 341.

Robert L. Dickman ● Director, Department of Family Medicine, Mount Sinai Medical Center, University Circle, Cleveland, Ohio 44106.

groups and health care providers dedicated to developing new models of delivery in this country.

On the other hand, the notion of the right to health care has recently been subjected to varied and often critical analyses on a variety of levels. Physicians—concerned about the practical application of the concept within a complex delivery system, its effect on their professional lives, and even on the liberty of their patients—have questions, about its legitimacy.[3,4] Philosophers and legal thinkers have also subjected the notion to rigorous analyses in order to unpack some of the basic moral principles (if any) from which it derives and to comprehend how it might be applied within the context of any or all health care delivery systems.[5-7] Norman Daniels, for example, in a preliminary essay on the right to health care, states that "we are justified in claiming a right to health care only if it is derivable from an acceptable general theory of justice."[8] In a fairly thorough look at one such distributive theory (Rawls's) Daniels initially finds no such clear basis for the claim to a right to health care. By scrutinizing Rawls's notion of *justice as fairness,* Daniels means to "show how far we are from being able to derive rights to health care from even most sympathetic theoretical frameworks."[9] After carefully ex-

[3]Robert M. Sade, "Medical Care as a Right: A Refutation." *New England Journal of Medicine,* CCLXXXV (Dec. 2, 1971), 1288–92.

[4]Mark Siegler, "A Right to Health Care: Ambiguity, Professional Responsibility, and Patient Liberty," *Journal of Medicine and Philosophy,* IV (1979), 148.

[5]Charles Fried, "Rights and Health Care—Beyond Equity and Efficiency," *New England Journal of Medicine,* CCXCIII (July 31, 1975), 241–46.

[6]Robert M. Veatch, "What Is a 'Just' Health Care Delivery?" *Ethics and Health Policy,* edited by Robert Veatch and Roy Branson (Cambridge, Mass.: Ballinger, 1976), pp. 127–36.

[7]K. Arrow, "Uncertainty and the Welfare Economics of Medical Care," *American Economic Review,* LIII (1963) 941–73.

[8]Norman Daniels, "Rights to Health Care and Distributive Justice: Programmatic Worries," *Journal of Medicine and Philosophy,* IV (1979), 174–91.

[9]Ibid.

ploring a number of strategies open to those wishing to apply Rawls's theory to health care and rejecting them all, Daniels concludes that it appears "surprisingly if not impossibly difficult to flesh out that right within a framework of a theory that ought to be amenable to incorporating it."[10] Although not subjecting the theories of libertarianism or utilitarianism to similar analyses, Daniels suggests that a clear derivation of the right-to-health-care claim from those theories would be equally if not more difficult. For him, further analysis of the nature of health care as a social good will be necessary in order to lead to a resolution of some of the distributive issues. In addition, these kinds of difficulties with the notion of the right to health care can pose a serious problem for health care reformers: if indeed change in the health care system seeks its ultimate (moral) justification within the tenuous principle of the right to health care or in its often unclear application, then redress may be difficult to conceptualize and even harder to obtain.[11]

It is the purpose of this essay to consider this problem from yet another perspective and thereby to suggest that—given at least a willingness if not an obligation to provide some health care services to all—there is a moral duty to deliver them in a way that argues for a very *basic* change in one significant part of our health care system. In order to advance this idea, I shall first have to describe a basic problem within an existing segment of the U.S. health care system. Second, I will need to invoke a moral principle that would seem pertinent to this problem and show what may be special about health care goods that allows for moral arguments on their behalf. Third, I will have to impose a method for applying that principle to the problem under discus-

[10]Ibid.

[11]I assume that those concerned with distributive questions about health are searching for some foundation upon which to either change or justify the present system.

sion. Finally, to make this issue concrete, I will present a real-life example of a health care delivery model whose moral worth may be based on the premises I will set forth.

It must be made clear at the outset that the argument rehearsed in this paper will not, in and of itself, necessitate full equity in or even equal access to health care services. I seek, rather, a method to redress one major problem in our present delivery system through the application of a first-order moral principle upon which most can agree. This kind of analysis will not satisfy those who seek a methodology for determining exactly what services we are to provide within a just delivery system. On the other hand, I mean to show that this perspective may enable us to approximate closely a model of health service that most would consider equitable.

I

The health care industry, with projected and annual expenses of over 200 billion[12] (approximately 9% of the gross national product), is a complex web of public and private providers, institutions, and assorted overseers that defies simplistic characterization or description. The pluralistic nature of the system makes it difficult to distill its problems and necessitates study by economists, politicians, epidemiologists, and many others even to begin to delineate the many facets of its major weaknesses and deficiencies adequately. Problems of access, quality assurance, and cost and efficiency of services are but a few of the issues of great concern to students of the U.S. health care system. One

[12]Joseph A. Califano, Jr., *Remarks before the Association of American Medical Colleges*, New Orleans, Louisiana, Oct. 24, 1978 (Washington, D.C.: U.S. Government Printing Office, 1978).

general but complex problem of significant proportions and of particular concern to the purposes of this essay has to do with the nature of municipal hospital-based services now available to the economically and socially disadvantaged living in large urban areas (more than 30 million of our citizens).[13]

The history of health care of the poor in America can be traced to colonial times.[14] Many colonial towns hired physicians to provide services to the poor and, in fact, hospitals developed around this concern. Both the Charity Hospital in New Orleans and the Philadelphia General (the two oldest hospitals in America) evolved from almshouses and were designed to provide services for the poor and the homeless.[15] Physicians, in return for providing free care to the poor in the hospital dispensaries, were given the privilege of bringing their apprentices on rounds, thus enabling them to obtain direct "hands-on" clinical experience. Thus it is clear (at least in historical terms) that our society has always been (charitably) prepared to provide at least some health care services to all.

Throughout the twentieth century, physicians continued to provide this kind of free care to the medically indigent in our large cities. Seriously ill poor patients were admitted to both municipal and private hospitals as "service cases," were supervised by attendings, and were cared for by students and house officers. Hospital outpatient departments, targeted for use by the poor, developed rapidly over the last hundred years, with care being provided by voluntary attendings, students, and house officers. The entire spectrum of emergency and ambulatory services was usually available in these settings.

[13]K. Davis, "Medical Payments and Utilization of Medical Services by the Poor," *Inquiry*, XIII (1976), 122–34.
[14]John Duffy, *The Healers: The Rise of the Medical Establishment* (New York: McGraw Hill, 1976), p. 57.
[15]Ibid. p. 31.

The introduction of Medicare and Medicaid in 1965, designed to enfranchise the poor medically did little to alter this basic urban delivery model—although, for the first time, hospitals and doctors were reimbursed for these services and the poor were increasing their use of the system.[16] These federal and state insurance programs, although intended to enable the poor to gain access to the private sector, were far from successful. Although some integration did take place, physicians were unable (because of time constraints) or unwilling (because of difficulty in getting appropriate and timely reimbursement) to accommodate all of the newly enfranchised patients, and the barriers to full health care in the private sector continued. A large proportion of city residents, therefore, continued to use the services of the hospital clinics and wards, as their ancestors had done for the last hundred years.

It is important to delineate why some may consider this hospital-based delivery system for our urban poor to be inferior to other models. Since most hospitals in the system are teaching institutions, the technical amount of care available is often similar to (and sometimes better than) that in the private sector. An acutely ill patient, for example, is rarely if ever denied care. Supervising (teaching) attendings bring their considerable expertise and clinical acumen to each case; students and house officers, if inexperienced, are bright and conscientious. The diagnosis and treatment given in both the inpatient and outpatient settings are often of good technical quality. Nevertheless, major deficiencies exist within this model, at least in the minds of some.

The problems in the hospital-based delivery system for the urban poor can be identified on a number of levels and go beyond the usual boundaries of technical medical care. Deficiencies can

[16]Elizabeth A. Skimmer *et al.*, "Use of Ambulatory Health Services by the Near Poor," *American Journal of Public Health*, LXVIII (December 1978), 1195–1201.

be described first in terms of the lack of nonmedical amenities that other patients have come to expect. Clinic waiting rooms are often dreary, with long rows of benches on which ill and anxious clients must wait. Many clinics have no functioning appointment system and work on a "first come, first served" basis, with the result that many patients come early, prepared to spend the day. One recent study pointed to an average wait of over three hours for a physician encounter of about 7½ minutes![17]

Once inside the examining rooms, patients encounter further difficulties. They are often seen by residents anxious to return to the drama of inpatient medicine or by attendings merely putting in their time and available to these patients for only a few hours a week. Further, in teaching centers (most large municipal hospitals), patients, without their consent, may be subjected to numerous examinations or intimate questioning by inexperienced medical students. For example, doctors in training are often taught the technique of pelvic examination on clinical patients, and one such patient may undergo several examinations during a single encounter.

These kinds of problems also exist on the inpatient side. "Service cases" are relegated to the least attractive quarters and sometimes placed in large wards. Even where the accommodations are noticeably improved, students and house officers—often with no previous knowledge of the patients—provide most of the care. The patients are subjected to a host of unfamiliar faces and repeated examinations.

Most importantly, patients in this system fail to develop a continuing and meaningful relationship with a single health care provider. In the clinic they most content with turnover in house officers and students as well as with attendings, who are available

[17]F. A. Finnerty, Jr., E. C. Mattie, and F. A. Finnerty III, "Hypertension in the Inner City: I. Analysis of Clinic Dropouts," *Circulation*, LXVII (1973), 76–78.

only during certain hours. In addition, the young physicians in these settings, forced to deal with large numbers of patients whose cultural and social mores are vastly different from their own, tend to be judgmental and even critical of their clientele. Because they are in the clinic for such short periods of time, the professionals rarely get an opportunity to know their patients except in a most superficial way. When patients require help during evenings and weekends, they are instructed to use the hospital emergency services, where a whole new set of providers is encountered. When admitted to the hospital, patients are not usually cared for by the clinic doctor and hence encounter further fragmentation, sometimes during the same episode of illness. Patients admitted toward the end of any month, for instance, will see a new group of students, residents, and attendings on the first of the new month and be forced to submit to further workups and additional probing.

To be sure, this picture of inner-city health care is not universally representative. A number of hospitals and neighborhood health centers have started to correct these kinds of deficiencies. Few of these, however, are able to retain for very long fully trained physicians prepared to make these practices their full-time career. Although some of these health centers provide patients with more comfortable and dignified surroundings, they are still in a minority and usually fail (for lack of funds—especially in the last few years) to redress all the basic difficulties to which I have alluded. In particular, very few of these centers have been able to solve the problems of continuity of care when the patients require hospitalization.

Delineating deficiencies of a health care system in these terms suggests that we must consider more than the technical components of care when we evaluate any delivery model. The kinds of problems I have described within the municipal hospital delivery system seem to be concerned with the way people (both consumers and providers) are made to *feel* within that setting. The fundamental deficiency of that system lies in its failure to respect the autonomy of its clients and to create an atmosphere that allows them to maintain their self-respect.

The fact of being ill poses the greatest threat to the integrity and freedom of any individual.[18] Ill or injured patients sense a certain disruption of the rhythm of life and subsequently become constantly preoccupied with their health problems. This preoccupation, along with pain and/or suffering, prevents them from making unencumbered choices about important aspects of their lives. Almost thirty years ago, Parsons delineated the "sick role" and pointed to how it can absolve one from many of life's responsibilities.[19] This diminished responsibility clearly diminishes the individual's moral agency as well. The "fact of illness"[20] and its subsequent threat to personhood is what usually leads people to seek access to the health care system. If, during that encounter (no matter how technically competent), the already seriously threatened autonomy of the patient becomes compromised even further by the very nature of the delivery system, a moral violation can be perceived to exist.

It is this essential ontological assault produced by illness or injury that allows for moral arguments on behalf of health care services and therefore makes them different from other goods. There are at least two other arguments on behalf of singling out health services as special. Daniels claims that certain health services are unique because they are a necessary condition for future opportunity.[21] Gutmann argues that pain (and suffering) alone

[18]Edmund D. Pellegrino, "Towards a Reconstruction of Medical Morality: The Primacy of the *Act* of Profession and the *Fact* of Illness," *Journal of Medicine and Philosophy,* IV (March), 1979.

[19]T. Parsons, *The Social System* (New York: The Free Press), 1951.

[20]Pellegrino, "Towards a Reconstruction of Medical Morality."

[21]N. Daniels, "Health-Care Needs and Distributive Justice," *Philosophy and Public Affairs,* X (1981), 146–79.

may be sufficient reason for singling out as special the goods that are concerned with alleviating or preventing it.[22] It appears then, without fleshing out any of these arguments, that there are a number of reasons to lay claim to the intuitive notion that health care goods have different value than other commodities and that second-class (tourist) air travel or second-class (bleacher) seats at a ballgame are less of a problem than second class (clinic) medicine. In this last case, respect for persons seems worthy of primary consideration.

Clinic care for the poor violates the principle of respect for persons in two general ways. First, because care in this setting is often perceived by both clients and providers as charity, the former have a hard time laying claim to their rights to respect and autonomy and thereby diminish their own self-respect. Further, since some providers (house staff) perceive their work in primary care as an "add-on" to their training, they will be less capable of acknowledging the rights of their clients. Other providers (attendings) who view their work with clinic patients as beneficent will at best be paternalistic in regard to their interactions with them. Second, the nature of the milieu in which this care is provided makes it difficult if not impossible for professionals to act in ways that show respect for their patients. There are a number of specific ways in which this circumstance is produced: the existence of undignified or dehumanizing surroundings, long waiting lines, groups of students learning on a patient without that patient's informed consent, and the provision of care in a hurried and fragmented way or in a manner that causes the intimacies of the human condition to be laid bare abruptly, discontinuously, and out of context with the rest of the patient's personal circumstances. It is not the surroundings them-

[22]Amy Gutmann, "For and Against Equal Access to Health Care," *Milbank Memorial Fund Quarterly/Health and Society,* LIX (1981) 542–60.

selves that *de novo* violate any moral principle. Rather, they make it possible for violations to take place in face-to-face encounters. In addition, patients forced to sit in dreary surroundings and then seen quickly by different providers who are rarely fully informed of their problems will have a hard time laying claim to their own self-respect. Clearly, the external environment only makes possible these occurrences. Therefore, as I will show later, improvements in that environment will not necessarily ensure respect for persons.

Thus, by being perceived as charity and practiced in an environment that allows for the dehumanization of patient interaction, health care for the urban poor violates human dignity and compromises personhood because it fails to treat individuals as ends in themselves, seeing them instead as a means to some further end. In that sense, clinical care for the poor has as its roots the violation of a basic, unconditional moral rule.

II

I have thus far attempted to describe a problem in one component of our delivery system in terms that may allow us to look to a basic moral principle as a foundation for redress. The problem in health care for inner-city poor has many facets but appears quite clearly to represent an encroachment on the autonomy and self-respect of patients. I have also shown that the fact of illness and the explicit nature of the health care encounter already tend to strip responsibility from individuals, so that further violations will be particularly devasting.

If we are willing to accept the principle of respect for persons (and it appears hard not to), we can develop a basis for discovering how we ought to act in regard to the delivery of health care services to any group of people. Unlike the principles of equity, liberty, or utility, which are often invoked to justify health policy, this moral principle seems less subject to rational critique. It therefore seems a more solid foundation on which to seek reform. Furthermore, a careful application of this principle can lead to significant and at times profound changes for certain groups in the health care system.

The moral principle of respect for persons contains within it at least two concepts about which there may be a certain tension that is not easily resolved. That is, such a principle implies both the acknowledgment of the individual's right to self-determination and the responsibility of others always to treat people with respect. To be sure, both components will need application within health care settings, but it is the latter notion upon which this particular essay has chosen to focus. Autonomy and its derivative notion of informed consent appears to be an issue in all health care encounters; although it may be a necessary prerequisite for respect for persons, it is beyond the scope of this essay.[23] The particular nature of the health care received by many of the urban poor in inner-city hospitals clearly appears to violate the principle of never treating people as means but always as ends in themselves. The moral worthiness of any health care system must be measured at least in terms of the degree to which it maintains this concept of respect for persons.

III

In order to develop an ethical basis for redness of this major qualitative deficiency in the delivery of health services to the

---

[23]The achievement of informed consent, is, like many other things, more of a problem for the poor than for others in our society. Recent data have shown, for example, that doctors provide more information to middle-class patients than they do to poor ones. Cf. David S. Brody, "The Patient's Role in Clinical Decision-Making," *Annals of Internal Medicine*, XCIII (1980) 718–22.

urban poor, we will need to do more than simply invoke the principle of respect for persons and the necessity for its strict application in the health care setting. A reemphasis of the health care provider's duty to treat persons with respect may be necessary, but this in itself is not sufficient to bring about reform within the system. The task of putting this principle of respect for persons in operation within a health service can be approached in two ways. One might be to detail either directly or indirectly all those things about an existent or proposed system that might be considered actual or potential violations of the principle. This delineation would then have to be followed up with a program designed specifically to avoid or correct such problems.

In many respects, this kind of planning seems sensible. The kinds of problems described in an earlier section of this essay can easily be corrected. Waiting times, patient satisfaction, and even continuity of care are all measurable and can be used as yardsticks for evaluating compliance with the principle I have outlined. On the other hand, this approach to ensuring the moral worth of any health service has a major flaw. That is, any of these measurements assures respect for persons only indirectly. It is not hard to conceive of a delivery model with, for example, that has short waiting times and a comfortable waiting room but yet fails to treat its clients with respect.

Other violations of the principle that are more difficult to catalogue may exist within the system. As we have previously suggested, the ultimate realization of this principle involves a change in both awareness and behavior. Any assessment of this principle must be understood within that context.

It will be necessary, therefore, to consider a secondary rule that when interposed between this primary principle and the realities we are concerned with, will provide a better strategy with which to measure reform. Put in its first-order and most literal way, this formulation might read: "A health care system maintains respect for persons if reasonable people with other available options choose to use it and continue to use it over time."

The ability of a health care delivery model to recruit and retain clients against a set of alternatives can serve as measure of the moral worth of the system in the sense I have described. It is important, however, to stress that these judges must be neither captive nor jaded. Thus, we could not consider reasonable those whose personal freedoms haye been stripped away in so many other ways that further encroachments, as within the health care setting, will not be accurately perceived. On the other hand, we would also not consider reasonable those elite few who might consider the presence of expensive art in the waiting room of a health center as a sign of the practitioners' respect for persons.

We may come to understand this notion better in practical terms by way of the following hypothetical situation. Suppose for a moment that, being impressed with the particular part of the problem in urban health care I have described, you wanted to advance reform in a way that would allow you to build on the moral foundation I have outlined. Since you are knowledgeable about planning and implementing health care delivery models, you set about creating a setting (to deliver a predetermined quantum of technical medical care) that to the best of your abilities, will be designed to hold sacred the personal autonomy and dignity of your clients. No matter how ambitious your project, you would probably have some difficulty in determining whether you were successful (in the context of respect for persons) without resorting to the use of reasonable judges. One way might be to see whether you yourself (presumably a reasonable judge) would find the service acceptable and, infact, would actually use the facilities you have created. Another might be to see whether people with the ability and mobility *to choose* alternatives would, geography permitting, in fact avail themselves of these services. The creation of a health service exclusively for a disenfranchised (captive) group with essentially no available alternatives will in and of itself not ensure the service's moral worth. One would always be hard put to justify the service morally without subjecting it to the judgment of some who will go elsewhere if their freedom and sense of self-worth is too severely bruised. In this sense the behavior of the inner-city poor client may not be a fair test of the adequacies of the service. (This failure to judge as a reasonable person in no way suggests that such individuals are always incapable of knowing when violations of their dignity have taken place. Rather, it implies that since no other options may be open to them or they may have become "immune" to these encroachments, their continued use of the service may not *in and of itself* be convincing proof of the adequacy of the service in the qualitative sense I have been addressing.)

Further, in order for this application to have meaning in the experiment we have described, we have to assume (and I think we can in the pluralistic system in which we live) that there are a variety of (reasonable) health care options from which our reasonable person can make a choice. Clearly, if all of the available options were either identical to or worse than the one being examined, any choice of it by these judges would have little meaning. We then come to see that a necessary condition for this experiment is a pluralistic system of health care with the existence of alternative and morally viable options. In fact, ensuring dignity and freedom in a universal and uniform system through this "test" would not be practical, as the individual's decision to remain within it would mean little. (This should be taken as an argument not against a national health system but against the application of this *particular principle* in that system.) Further consideration suggests at least two significant problems.

First, retention of clients with options does not in and of itself guarantee that all patients in the system will be treated in a way that maximizes their dignity. It is not hard to imagine a model where certain patients are treated optimally and others less so. (This is particularly true when the former are either easily identifiable or voice their concerns or complaints openly.) One could then construct a service within this framework that provided both equitable and inequitable service under one roof.

We will need to make two suppositions in order to preclude this "worse case." The first is that changes in the system designed to pass the test will clearly be applicable to all. (Continuity of care, an on-call system, and comfortable facilities are but a few examples.) Second is that workers in this system will not be constantly "shifting gears" depending on the particular client. Seeing people on time, treating them with respect, and minimizing affronts to their dignity becomes an approach within an entire system rather than a constantly changing phenomenon. An atmosphere that satisfies the reasonable judge is more likely than not to spill over to all involved.

A second potential problem with this methodology is that we can imagine a situation (particularly where we have not assumed equity) in which all the alternatives will simply be better or offer more than in the one under scrutiny. Would the tendency of even reasonable judges to "trade up" in that case to taken as an absolute indictment of the present system? It is in regard to this problem that we are forced to consider quantitative issues in our argument. If the alternatives offer significantly more than our system provides, then all the judges will trade up. Within the framework of our analysis, such behavior would discredit the system under scrutiny, and well it should. On the other hand, we will have to presume that while small specific differences (increases in services offered or nicer facilities) may attract a few such judges, not all will perceive them as better. Health care goods differ from other commodities in that their value in most people's eyes is rarely perceived on a fine scale. Assuming a satisfactory relationship with the doctor and treatment that maintains respect, patients will rarely seek alternatives unless they have an unusual need or a desire for specific services. On the basis of past experience, we know that such needs will be the exception rather than the rule. Nevertheless, this kind of analysis forces us to consider quantity as well as quality. In order to maintain autonomy, it appears that any delivery system must possess a basic minimum of services and deliver them in a minimally respectful way. We will attempt to define this minimum at the conclusion of the paper.

To summarize, the best test of whether a health care service has indeed addressed this qualitative problem (fundamental to the hospital-based care of the inner city poor) is the continued participation of a group of clients who have chosen the service over others. Thus a new delivery model that is available to those formerly relegated to the clinic will remain morally worthy (i.e., consistent with the imperative of respect for persons) as long as it is able to attract people with the option of choosing alternative forms.

IV

I want now to cite a specific real-life example of this kind of approach to reform in the health care system. By doing so, I mean to suggest that there are examples of redress that can be well grounded in the moral position I have developed and can serve in that sense as an example of what we ought to be doing on a larger scale. Although not entirely unique, this case study provides us with concrete evidence that reform is indeed realistic while remaining consistent with the proposals I have put forth. To be sure, one does not need lofty moral arguments to realize that this system is better than the one I have discussed. By describing it I mean to show that it is not only intuitively better but also morally better and therefore can be advocated in more categorical terms.

Prior to 1973, a community hospital in Rochester, New York, operated an outpatient department in the manner I have described at the outset of this essay. Located on the fringes of the inner city in a working-class neighborhood, the clinic served patients primarily from the inner-city area. Clients were seen by house officers, students, and "voluntary" attendings in a generally dreary environment with little continuity of care. A health planner and a physician, concerned about this problem, developed a program that was intended, both ideologically and literally, to close the clinic. Using the resources already available for the health care of the inner-city poor (Medicaid) and realizing that the location of the hospital was such that it could potentially attract a wider socioeconomic spectrum of patients, these planners developed and implemented the concept of a hospital-based group practice to be located in a doctor's office across from the hospital. The planners called on some physicians with busy practices in the community to join the group; they also recruited new M.D.s for the program. The practice was envisioned to care for the entire clinic population, while also attracting *new* clients to the service who might not normally use the typical outpatient department. The planners reasoned that since the financial success of their program depended on their ability to recruit and retain patients who had other options for health care, they would then be obligated to assure a certain quality within that system.

All the former clinic patients as well as new inner-city clients were incorporated into this new model, but they represented only 40% of the total patient population. These people were now followed in the context of a group practice and became identified with a single health care provider. The care they received was in no way distinguishable from that obtained by the clients who continued to choose this setting over options available within the traditional private sector. Since the financial success of the practice required recruitment and retention of financially viable clients, a certain quality of care (both institutionally and interpersonally) was ensured. Patients waited in small, pleasantly decorated waiting rooms and an appointment system was scrupulously adhered to. Student and resident physicians were incorporated into the practice for blocks of time and in a fashion that would not be offensive to any of the patients. In addition to having obvious intuitive appeal, this kind of major reform can be solidly grounded ethically and need not to rely exclusively on principles of distributive justice or equity for its moral appeal. Rather than addressing itself to a quantitative allocation of goods and services, the practice radically altered the milieu in which these services were developed. The success of the project in a moral sense (and in a financial one) was measured by the ability to retain in the practice those with options to leave and can be viewed as consistent with the principle of respect for persons.

V

It has been the purpose of this essay to suggest (in a preliminary fashion) that there may be moral obligations in the delivery of health services that depend on implementing respect for persons, a basic moral imperative upon which most can agree. It needs to be reiterated, however, that in no way does this kind of argument tell us how much to provide to any group, nor does it preclude some inequities in health care services. In order for this proposal to have practical import we must assume a willingness (not necessarily an obligation) to provide some services to those presently not capable of purchasing them directly. Assuming this, our analysis requires the provision of such services in a specific way.

Charles Fried, in an earlier essay, argues for the notion of a "decent minimum"[24] of health services that he claims should be available to all regardless of circumstances. He fails, however, to provide us with any truly concrete notion of what he really means and states "that the notion of minimum health care, which it does make sense for our society to recognize as a right, is itself an unstable and changing notion."[25] What we mean to suggest is that the notion of "minimum health care" in a quantitative sense may be unstable and continuously changing; respect for persons within that minimum remains a moral absolute. As long as our society allows for *any* health services to be available to the poor, it becomes morally necessary to deliver them in a fashion that minimizes violations of the dignity of moral agents. In our analysis, there would need to be at least two necessary components of a decent minimum. First (and most important), a continuous relationship with a competent provider and, second, an environment that does not allow for loss of respect.

Regardless of quantity, these aspects of a delivery model can lead to reforms in health care area that have strong appeal to those of us concerned about the personal quality of services we are now providing to our medically indigent. Although clearly not an argument on behalf of equal health services for all, compliance with this standard will (as a side benefit) create more equity in the system than now exists.

It may also be argued that in no way has this strategy guaranteed a standardized or acceptable level of technical medical competence in any one delivery model. By focusing our discussion on the area of human dignity and respect for persons and designating lay people as judges, may we possibly certify a system that delivers dignified and respectful care in an incompetent

[24]Charles Fried, "Analysis of 'Equality' and 'Rights' in Medical Care," *Hastings Center Report*, VI (February, 1976).
[25]Ibid.

fashion? Are we in essence allowing for the possibility of medically substandard but attractively packaged health services? The same can be said for a health care system that seeks its justification on the basis of equity of fairness. We can imagine a system that fairly and equitably provides substandard care to all. Similarly, proponents of equity in health care services will either have to assume technical competence or argue for it in some other way than on the basis of a strict appeal to that principle alone.

We will need, I think, a whole new set of arguments to deal with this problem, which must be approached not from the view of the kinds of services we can provide but rather from a foundation of medical morality and the medical competence inherent in the "act of profession" by any health care provider. The moral obligation of technical competence may also have to be concerned with the notion of respect for persons. (One might add that lying is an obvious violation of respect for persons, and that falsely professing competence is one form of lying.) Pellegrino, in a major essay, begins to lay the foundation for this kind of approach.[26]

In conclusion, in this essay we have attempted to detail a problem in our present health care system that some may want to redress by invoking a claim to the right to health care based on principles of justice and/or equity. By focusing the analysis on the principle of respect for persons, we are obligated in general ways to upgrade the level of service we are providing to our inner city poor. By measuring the degree to which this principle is maintained by the behavior of reasonable judges, we begin to flesh out a decent minimum in terms other than those considered by Fried. Nevertheless, this kind of analysis will, in the end, never tell us just how much or what kind of health care services to provide.

By the same token, those who argue for equal access to health

---

[26]Pellegrino, "Towards a Reconstruction of Medical Morality."

care face similar problems. In her paper on this topic, Gutmann is quick to point out that "the equal access principle does not establish whether a society must provide a particular medical treatment or health care benefit to its needy members."[27] Putting the principle of respect for persons into operation can allow for inequities only within the context of that rule. As we have shown, these inequities will either reflect desires (fine art in the waiting room or cosmetic surgery or unusual needs. When considering such desires or unusual needs, equity cannot exist.

Neither the principle of equity nor respect for persons will help us to determine just what quantities of unusual services we will provide to any or all in a society. In a nation that values liberty and has limited economic resources, all competing for a variety of programs, decisions regarding how much health care to deliver will never satisfy everyone.

[27]Gutmann, "For and Against Equal Access," pp. 542–60.

7

Jerry Avorn

Needs, Wants, Demands, and Interests
THEIR INTERACTION IN MEDICAL PRACTICE AND HEALTH POLICY

Health and Needs

The Hastings Center Working Group on Ethics and Health Policy began its work in the late 1970s at a time when it still seemed plausible for adult men and women to sit together and discuss what goals the American health care system might set for itself and how we as a nation might most justly accomplish these goals. Now, in the early 1980s, in the midst of an unprecedented retrenchment in health care programs and other public services, it seems somewhat naive to address these questions with anything but a heavy sense of irony. Nonetheless, it is still useful to consider the relationship between health needs, health care wants, and interests in the formulation and delivery of medical services with the hope and expectation that within the next few years the

Jerry Avorn ● Assistant Professor of Social Medicine and Health Policy, Division on Aging, Harvard Medical School, and attending physician, Beth Israel Hospital, Boston, Massachusetts 02115.

allocation of resources to meet human needs once again will become an important part of the national agenda.

The World Health Organization (WHO) in its well-known definition of health as the goal of medical care[1] was certainly correct in attempting to relate the presence or absence of somatic disease to larger concerns, such as the relationship of the individual to the environment and to society. Yet, as Daniel Callahan has noted,[2] broadening the concept of health to include not just the absence of disease but also the presence of complete physical, mental, and social well-being may sometimes obscure more issues than it illuminates. One suspects that, had the WHO definition been formulated in the late 1960s instead of the late 1940s, a notion of health would have emerged that comprised "complete physical, mental, social, *and spiritual* well-being." (While appealing as a state, such definitions burden the medical care system with so many additional responsibilities and considerations as to make it vulnerable to collapse under the extra weight.) Clearly, one's physical state is inextricably linked to one's social condition and one's emotional status. Nonetheless, this essay will be limited to the experience, assessment, and management of those medical problems that are primarily somatic in nature. Analogies to emotional, social, or cosmic states may inadvertently suggest themselves, but the focus will remain the *physical* component of health and disease.

Health services theory and research are replete with heroic attempts to define a "gold standard" of physical health toward which any rational policy or system would aim. Confining ourselves to the physical component of health, we can, for the purposes of the present discussion, define good physical health as

[1]World Health Organization, "The Constitution of the World Health Organization," *WHO Chronicle* I (1947), 29.
[2]Daniel Callahan, "The WHO Definition of 'Health,' " *Hastings Center Studies,* I (1973), 77–87.

the condition of an organism's body that enables it to approach optimal age-specific physical functioning. This somewhat simple-minded definition of health will make possible an examination of the relationships among needs, demands, and interests in medical care.

Toward a Definition of Needs

When the definition of good health is temporarily restricted to its physical component, a scientific definition of health needs becomes possible. For the already healthy person, the concept of a health service need is conceptually straightforward but operationally still somewhat confusing. The randomized clinical trial works well in determining whether or not a particular preventive health intervention, such as a biannual Pap test or annual sigmoidoscopic examination, makes a difference in the prevention of disease. That such issues are still a source of great confusion relates to two factors: (1) the sluggishness with which medical research has addressed questions of prevention and large-scale epidemiologic trials and (2) the clouding of issues that has resulted from the injection of nonscience-based concerns (such as how medical services are reimbursed) into consideration of these questions. Nonetheless, the problem remains simple in theory.

For the sick patient, definition of genuine health care needs is likewise theoretically straightforward, though it is a painstaking and arduous task to put this approach into operation. Once again, the instrument needed to distinguish necessary from irrelevant medical interventions is the controlled clinical trial, ideally a randomized double-blind trial. The entire history of clinical research, particularly in the last thirty years, can be seen as the laborious implementation of this approach to distinguish geniune from ineffectual interventions in health care.[3] Whether steroids are useful in the treatment of hepatitis (and which kinds of hepatitis), whether pneumococcal vaccine can prevent pneumonia (and in whom), whether coronary artery bypass surgery prolongs life—all these questions can be answered by appropriately designed and conducted controlled clinical trials, though the process takes years to complete for each question. This approach is what separates contemporary physicians (in many instances) from witch doctors, and it is the reason that we no longer make much use of leeches.

It is by now apparent that this reduction of health care needs to a simple technical level of "promoting optimal physical functioning of the organism" has, in the course of narrowing of the terms of the discussion, excluded from consideration some interesting and important questions. For instance, is hemodialysis a health care "need" for a 90-year-old man with kidney failure who has been severely demented for several years, is both paralyzed and incontinent, and has developed widespread, painful terminal cancer? Using our definition, the answer is yes: in order to optimize the level of this patient's physical functioning, under our definition the patient physically *needs* dialysis; his level of physiological functioning will undoubtedly deteriorate and death will no doubt ensue more rapidly without this treatment. However, this is not to say that such a patient *should* be dialyzed. Other considerations from the realm of ethics,[4] or even of economics[5] may become injected into the clinical decision mak-

---

[3]A. L. Cochrane, *Effectiveness and Efficiency: Random Reflections on Health Services* (London: Nuffeld Provincial Hospitals Trust, 1972).

[4]Arthur L. Caplan, "Kidneys, Ethics, and Politics: Policy Lessons of the ESRD Experience," *Journal of Health Politics, Policy, and Law*, VI (1981), 488–503.

[5]Richard A. Rettig, "The Policy Debate on Patient Care Financing for Victims of End-Stage Renal Disease," *Law and Contemporary Problems*, XL (1977), 196–230.

ing process so as to override considerations based solely on physiological need. Were that patient a member of my family or even me, I would certainly opt for no dialysis. The critical point in such a decision must not be made (as it often is) for the reason, "The patient does not need to be dialyzed." Rather, adhering to our admittedly simple-minded definition of health, we are forced to address the issues head-on and to be clear about when we are making a physiological statement as opposed to an ethical statement, or a cost-containment statement. Experience in a variety of clinical settings makes it clear that these languages are used interchangeably in such microallocation decisions all the time, doing considerable violence to the clarity of the discourse and often to the patients themselves. While bland and self-evident at first glance, the toned-down definition of medical "need" helps to clarify clinical decision making by separating out sick–well issues from right–wrong issues.

Demands Are Not Needs

Let us use next the term *want* to describe the subjective experience of a person who desires a particular intervention related to physical health. It is important to note that such a want may have nothing to do with an actual *need* for medical care, as will become apparent in the examples cited below. The subsequent communication of a health care want to someone in the health care delivery system transforms it into a *demand*. An important literature exists on the lack of identity between health care wants and health care demands. The perception of a desire for health services may never find expression because it is hampered by the constraints of poverty, racism, inaccessibility of medical services, or other causes of real or perceived disenfranchisement from the health care system. Thus, while all health care demands begin as wants, not all wants become translated into demands. Similarly, because wants can exist without needs and vice versa, the correlation between needs and demands becomes even more tenuous.

Some clinical examples may help to clarify these distinctions. In his classic study *The Health of Regionville*,[6] Koos described a number of situations that can be used to illustrate this terminology. One impoverished woman he interviewed suffered from uterine prolapse, an unsightly and uncomfortable condition in which the musculature of the pelvis no longer effectively contains the uterus and it sags out through the vaginal orifice. The woman was aware of the condition, wanted to have it corrected, but did not have the money for surgery. As a result, her health care want (in this case identical to her health care need) never became translated into a health care demand. (This example is instructive for those who attempt to assess needs for health care services by surveying the demands for same in any community.) Another woman experienced progressive swelling of her ankles and shortness of breath but attributed it to "growing old" and did not seek medical help. She apparently suffered from congestive heart failure, which might well have been treated with digitalis and/or diuretics, thus significantly improving her level of functioning. That is, her health care need was never perceived as a want and thus could not be translated into a demand, despite the fact that she suffered from a real and treatable medical problem. Such a failure to perceive health care needs is an important problem in clinical geriatrics. In this field, what Butler[7] has called "ageism" often causes the elderly, their families, and even their physicians

---

[6]Earl L. Koos, *The Health of Regionville* (New York: Columbia University Press, 1952).

[7]Robert N. Butler, *Why Survive? Growing Old in America* (New York: Harper & Row, 1975).

to misperceive real and often reversible pathological conditions as "just getting old."

Wants may not only be inappropriately absent, but also present yet physiologically "incorrect." That is, a patient with intestinal obstruction may want and demand an enema when what he really needs to prevent death is abdominal surgery. A completely different set of clinical problems arises when the opposite condition applies: wants and demands exist *beyond* actual physiological need. A patient with mild tension-related headaches may want a CAT scan but actually need just a few aspirins. In a controversial paper in the *New England Journal of Medicine* entitled "The Hateful Patient," Groves[8] describes a typology that includes overdemanding patients whose expectations for diagnosis and therapy exceed their actual somatic needs (though obviously not their psychiatric needs). Siegler[9] has also described such patients, who need little somatically but want and demand a great deal of their doctors. Again, this very common mismatch between needs on the one hand and wants on the other poses great peril for health care planners who base recommendations on the perceptions and actions of patients alone.

The Other Side of the Equation

Previous analyses of health care needs, such as those outlined by Donabedian,[10] address some of the concerns outlined above but often underestimate (or ignore entirely) the possibility that the *providers* of health care also bring their needs, wants, and

[8]James Groves, "Taking Care of the Hateful Patient," *New England Journal of Medicine*, CCXCVIII (April 20, 1978), 883–87.
[9]See Mark Siegler (Chapter 9) in this volume.
[10]Avedis Donabedian, *Aspects of Medical Care Administration* (Cambridge, Mass.: Harvard University Press, 1973).

demands to the clinical situation and that this may have an enormously important impact on the actual delivery of medical care. In much of the literature, the assumption appears to be that health care providers—whether they be doctors, nurses, hospital administrators, or third-party payers—approach the clinical encounter as if each individual or organization were a *tabula rasa* with no interest other than that of optimizing the patient's health. A wealth of evidence, from sociology,[11] economics,[12] and anthropology[13] indicates that this is clearly not the case. For the sake of simplicity, we need only consider the needs, wants, and demands of physicians, although analogous arguments can be made about these factors as they affect the behavior of nurses, hospitals, insurers, and other participants in the health care system.

The most self-evident need felt by physicians in relation to their patients is the need to make sick people well. Succeeding at this task gives most of us a sense of fulfillment and mastery that should, ideally, constitute most or all of the motivation that we bring to the doctor–patient encounter. However, a number of studies[14] have pointed out that physicians have other needs that often greatly affect this encounter and are much less directly related to the curing of disease. Prominent among these is the need to "have all the data." This need, which is a highly developed outgrowth of the schoolchild's need to get the right answer in class or on a test, is often manifested in the service of the patient but occasionally works against this goal. Students are selected for medical school based on their success at getting the

[11]Howard Becker *et al.*, *Boys in White: Student Culture in Medical School* (Dubuque, Iowa: William C. Brown, 1972).

[12]Victor Fuchs, *Who Shall Live? Health, Economics, and Social Choice* (New York: Basic Books, 1974).

[13]Claude Lévi-Strauss, *Structural Anthropology* (New York: Basic Books, 1963), chap. 9.

[14]Daniel H. Funkenstein, *Medical Students, Medical Schools, and Society During Five Eras* (Cambridge, Mass.: Ballinger Publishing Company, 1978).

right answer on a variety of tests throughout high school and college, and success in medical school is likewise achieved by those who are able to accumulate the most data in their preclinical and clinical training. A physician without data is like a sailboat without a sail, but this approach to the selection and training of physicians runs afoul when it is assumed that the sail can also serve as a rudder. In clinical practice, particularly in large teaching hospitals, the need to acquire data and find "the answer" is sometimes pursued beyond the interests of the patient. There is great deal of test-ordering behavior, invasive and noninvasive diagnostic procedures, and even occasional surgery primarily because of the need, selected for and intensified over the years in each of us, to find the right answer.

When clinical research is going on, of course, this need may be legitimate regardless of the irrelevance (not antagonism) of such behavior to the improvement of the patient's health status provided that the patient has been appropriately informed and consents to such additional investigation. Yet the mind set of research often carries over inappropriately to the bedside, bolstered by this particular orientation, and often with unfortunate results. Attempts to explain the sometimes irrational data mongering of physicians which do not take this very real need into account (and, for example, attribute such behavior to economic incentives exclusively) miss the point. Even physicians in prepaid practices, in which they may be insulated from concerns over profit, exhibit this tendency. Similarly, the concept of fear of malpractice ("defensive medicine") is likewise often advanced to explain such otherwise incomprehensible overordering of tests. Probably this too represents only a fraction of such behavior.

Other needs of physicians have been defined by psychologists and sociologists who have studied the development of physicians; these findings are quite germane to understanding the needs that are brought to the work of healing. The need to *control* is another example. The selection and training of physicians produces doctors who are highly motivated to control what is going on in patients' bodies, and also sometimes in their lives. This is generally not problematic, since sick people seek the help of a doctor in order that he or she may take charge of their disordered physiology and set it right. Such an approach is bolstered by the social relations that surround the doctor at every turn: we write "orders;" we are the "captains" of the health care "team." Yet the habit of control can run amok when it pushes aside other aspects of the physician's relationship with the patient (witness the difficulty so many physicians have in dealing with the "noncompliant" patient). In other cases, the need for control is expressed as attempts to "fix" things that do not, in fact, need to be fixed (e.g., the preoccupation with prescribing medication to treat trivially elevated levels of blood sugar or uric acid in otherwise healthy people). Again, to understand and ultimately correct this behavior, it is important to realize that much of it is merely an extension of an otherwise laudable need to take control over the illness we have been asked to exorcise.

A final need of physicians, often neglected in health services research, is their "activist orientation"—the tendency of physicians to prefer to take some sort of action rather than remain passive when faced with several equally effective ways of handling a clinical situation. It is the "Don't just stand there—*do* something" approach to illness. Most physicians are far more uncomfortable doing nothing than doing something, since the image of the effective physician is that of someone who *intervenes*. The problem, of course, occurs not when this is the most appropriate way of treating a given medical problem but rather when inaction is the wisest clinical course—a not uncommon situation in practice. As in the other characteristics outlined above, this predisposition is probably something which is selected for in medical school applicants, and it is certainly reinforced through the years

of medical school and especially internship and residency training.[15] And, like the others, it is quite distinct from the desire of
physicians to engage in therapeutic activities solely for the economic rewards such activity might produce—distinct from but
complementary to such a predisposition. The notion of an activist
orientation motivating physicians explains a great deal of the
frantic activity surrounding the care of the terminal cancer patient, activity that often ignores more humanistic "soft" concerns
about terminal care. To sit quietly with patients and help them
endure that which cannot be treated is a skill that comes only at
enormous psychological cost for many of us.

There are thus a series of needs experienced by most physicians as a result of their selection and training that are important
motivators of activity over and above the obvious need to make
sick patients healthy: the need to "find the right answer," the
need to be in control of the clinical situation, and the need to
engage in active diagnostics or therapeutic intervention. I will
not elaborate on the ways in which such needs are or are not
perceived and thus translated into wants and demands, as is the
case with the needs and wants of patients. However, it is worth
looking critically at another one of the physician's wants that has
an enormously important impact on the clinical process: the desire for remuneration.

In addition to the other motivations just noted, there is
considerable evidence that physicians frequently behave in a
manner that maximizes income, even when such behavior is not
necessarily part of a required therapeutic process. Specific examples that have been carefully documented in recent years include the higher rate of unnecessary surgery in situations in which
a fee-for-service reimbursement mechanism encourages surgeons

[15]Robert K. Merton, G. G. Reader, and P. L. Kendall, eds., *The Student Physician* (Cambridge, Mass.: Harvard University Press, 1957).

to operate, often when therapeutic indications are unimpressive;[16] the ritualistic and clinically useless nature of many aspects of the "routine annual physical," one of the more interesting religious practices of technological society;[17] and the astounding proliferation of laboratory tests of all kinds, which often generate the real economic payoff for physicians in private practice and hospital outpatient departments. Some of this activity may be explained in terms of the psychological needs of physicians. But it is striking to note the extent to which much of this unnecessary diagnostic and therapeutic activity drops off when the economic constraints of for-profit fee-for-service medicine are removed. Given that most of American health care still operates in this mode, a number of interesting problems emerge.

The physician's *want* is easily translated into a *demand* made on the patient, since the physician plays a commanding role in defining the agenda for many clinical interactions. However, the context in which the physician's wants are generally presented is that of the *patient's* health care *needs:* "Mrs. Smith, I think you need to come back to see me every six months for a Pap smear;" "Mr. Jones, you need to have that blood pressure of yours checked monthly." Thus, a want of the physician is translated into a demand on the patient, who, in turn, comes to believe that the activity discussed will address a real health care need and thus internalizes this want and transforms it into a demand made of the physician. The loop is complete in what must surely be one of the most complex forms of communication in all human intercourse. To the extent that the process reflects the patient's health care needs exclusively, the system works well; to the extent that other needs, wants, and demands are introduced, particu-

[16]Eugene Vayda, "A Comparison of Surgical Rates in Canada and in England and Wales," *New England Journal of Medicine*, CCLXXXIX (1973), 1224–29.

[17]Thomas L. Delbanco and William C. Taylor, The Periodic Health Examination," *Annals of Internal Medicine*, XCIII (1980), 773–75.

larly the want and demand for remuneration on the part of the physician independent of the patient's genuine health care needs, the system can generate a bewildering and ultimately very inefficient set of interactions that costs a great deal and benefits the patient little.

Dealing with Physicians' "Needs"

In attempting to relate the characteristics of patients and physicians, discussed above, to health care policy, one crucial point becomes apparent. The one person who is in the best position to judge whether a particular health care intervention, either diagnostic or therapeutic, will address a genuine health care need in a patient is the physician. The complexity of detail of modern medicine is simply too great to allow us to hope for very much sharing of the *technical* part of decision making with the patient in most instances, though the patient remains the "expert" in the values domain of clinical decision making. We have here a paradigm of the situation in which it is critical to separate out issues of expertise from issues of values or interests. An anonymous observer of human motivation summed up the situation succinctly a long time ago in the phrase, "The barber is not the person to ask if you need a haircut." In its purest form, the essence of the health maintenance organization (HMO) concept is precisely this: to uncouple the needs, wants, and demands of physicians from the clinical decision-making process except for the motivations associated with wanting to make the patient well. While regulation after the fact may be able to identify some instances of interventions designed primarily to benefit the doctor and not the patient, there is a much larger gray area of nonegregious activity (such as the frequency with which one schedules return visits for a patient with high blood pressure, or the plethora of tests scheduled as part of a routine annual physical examination) which are relatively immune from any kind of regulatory sanction. In my view, it is naive to expect a physician whose personal economic interest is involved to perform with optimal effectiveness and efficiency in such instances.

Lest the HMO concept appear too attractive, however, it is worth noting that it, too, can become the source of wants and demands on the part of the physician that do violence to the therapeutic encounter. To the extent that physicians are constrained by the HMO structure itself to underprovide services, an equally worrisome situation can come to exist. This situation is likeliest to occur in an HMO setting that is designed for profit and in which physicians or other stockholders benefit directly from any unexpended funds remaining at the end of a fiscal year. The "big business" approach that is said to have worked so well in the manufacturing of automobiles and other consumer goods cannot work effectively in health care. The difference in expertise in seller and consumer is too vast; the evidence suggest that patients do not behave like typical consumers in purchasing health care; and the consequences of incorrect "purchasing" or "selling" decisions are too extreme for a business model to apply.

Conclusions

It seems fair to conclude from the foregoing discussion that wants and demands on the part of either physicians or patients are unreliable guides to the provision of health care on either a micro (doctor–patient) or macro (policy) level. Aside from omitting many important health care needs from consideration and generating additional wants that do not in fact "need" to be met, the cost of such a haphazard system is astronomical. It is this last factor, that of costs out of control, that is currently forcing a reassessment of health care policy. A system of health care delivery based primarily on patients' legitimate health care needs can be constructed, although it flies in the face of most of the political economy of the American health care enterprise as it currently exists. As the exploding inefficiency and intolerable costs of our present approach force us to consider alternatives, it will also be important to consider the nonfinancial needs and wants of physicians discussed above, since they, too, significantly affect therapeutic decisions. At a time of dwindling resources and increasing scarcity, a more affordable and more equitable health care delivery system will also be a more austere one and will be hard for many physicians and patients to accept. However, the alternative of a minimally regulated system that provides essentially everything to the affluent and increasingly less to the poor is far less acceptable. The health care system that we will probably have by the end of this century was described (unintentionally) by Mick Jagger in the Rolling Stones' album *Let It Bleed:* "You can't always get what you want, but . . . you get what you need."[18] It's a catchy refrain that doctors and patients alike will probably find themselves dancing to before long.

[18]Mick Jagger *et al.*, *Let It Bleed*, (1969).

8

Mark Siegler

Physicians' Refusals of Patient Demands

AN APPLICATION OF MEDICAL DISCERNMENT

Introduction and Cases

This paper will present a series of cases indicating the range of problems that must be considered in determining whether physicians occasionally should refuse to accede to patients' demands.

Case 1

A middle-aged widow with chronic, treated hypertension had a slightly enlarged heart but showed no sign of functional heart impairment. This woman had worked hard for many years in order to support her two children, who had recently married and left home. She initially requested but soon demanded of the physician that she be declared physically disabled because of her high blood pressure and mild heart enlargement. She indicated that such disability would allow her to stop her arduous work

Mark Siegler ● Section of General Internal Medicine, Department of Medicine, University of Chicago–Pritzker School of Medicine, Chicago, Illinois 60637.

and to receive support from public funds as well as free medical care. She pointed out that her current medical insurance did not cover any outpatient costs and that the disability arrangement would permit her to receive better (or at least more complete) medical services than she could now afford. After reviewing the criteria of disability under the state statutes, her physician refused to declare her disabled.

Case 2

A middle-aged patient presented with a mild, asymptomatic iron-deficiency anemia of recent onset, The appropriate management of this condition should consist of a variety of tests—including blood tests, X-ray contrast studies, and possibly gastrointestinal endoscopy—all of which can be performed as outpatient procedures. The patient requested and soon demanded to be admitted to the hospital because this would be more convenient and because his insurance would cover only in-hospital costs. When his physician suggested that the insurance would cover only treatment and not diagnostic studies, the patient replied that this was a semantic quibble and that the physician could surely find a discharge diagnosis that the insurance company would pay for. The physician refused to admit the patient for the necessary studies and urged him to have such studies as an outpatient.

Case 3

A business executive, under considerable stress both at work and at home, for the first time in her life developed headaches. She was evaluated by her general internist and then referred to an excellent clinical neurologist. The neurologist and internist concurred that the quality, pattern, and type of pain and the total absence of neurological abnormalities suggested a diagnosis of tension headaches. The neurologist and internist were confident in their diagnosis and believed that no tests or X-rays studies were needed to confirm it. The patient requested but soon demanded a CAT scan from the internist. The patient had obviously read a considerable amount about CAT scans and argued as follows: "A small percent of treatable brain lesions [small tumors, AV malformations, and brain cysts] might be detected by this scan and might not be detected even by the best physicians and neurologists. The procedure is costly but not truly a scarce or limited resource, and in any event I volunteer to pay for the test rather than use my excellent private insurance plan. The risks of the procedure are very small [minimal radiation exposure and, remotely, an allergic reaction to the enhancing dye]." Consider two scenarios that might follow this demand:

1. The physician refused the patient's demand, confident in his diagnosis.
2. Although confident in his diagnosis, the physician finally acquiesced to the demand. The CAT scan was performed and its showings were entirely normal. The patient was temporarily reassured and the headaches diminished in intensity, but she returned three weeks later and complained that the headaches had not abated entirely. At that time, the patient demanded a repeat scan, arguing that the cause of her headaches (perhaps a tumor, etc.) may have been too small to have been detected in the original scan but now, three weeks later, the lesion might be detectable. At this point, the physician flatly refused to order a repeat scan.

Case 4

A university professor who was both physically and psychologically dependent on the consumption of 8 to 10 ounces of alcohol daily refused to admit that she was an alcoholic or had an "alcohol problem." She commuted by car to the university from the suburbs each day and only drank alcohol in the evening after returning home from work. She came to the physician's office complaining of inability to function effectively because of "insomnia" and initially requested and later demanded sleeping pills. She said: "I want sleeping pills so that I can sleep; then I will be able to work better and finish my book." After a frank discussion of the reasons for the decision, the physician refused to prescribe the sleeping pills.

Case 5

A 45-year-old athletic, nonsmoking university professor was well-known both to himself and to his primary physician of 10 years for his long-standing hypochondriacal symptoms, which usually appeared as abdominal or chest pain. Without informing his physician, he had started jogging 1½ years earlier and was now doing 10 to 12 miles five times a week. He came to the physician's office one day and said that his abdominal and chest pains had never really gone away, but when his jogging friends learned about them, they thought that he required a careful medical assessment to be "on the safe side." He requested an electrocardiogram and a multistage exercise test with thallium scanning. His physician agreed to the request and the results of both of these studies were entirely normal. The patient returned and requested, but soon demanded, a coronary angiogram. The patient argued that the only way to be certain that a 45-year-old male (even one without coronary risk factors) did not have coronary artery disease was to do the coronary angiogram. At this point, the physician refused to refer the patient to a cardiologist for the invasive catheterization study.

Case 5A. An obese middle-aged patient with chronic, asymptomatic liver disease requested and then demanded an ileojejunal bypass as treatment for his moderate, exogenous obesity. His physician refused to refer the patient to a surgeon and cited the risk of such an operation in patients with known liver disease.

Case 5B. A patient with mild nondisfiguring psoriasis of recent onset requested and then demanded methotrexate rather than standard, conventional, and less toxic treatment. After being informed of the risks of methotrexate, the patient insisted on the drug because it is relatively convenient to take and offers a high response rate. The physician refused to treat mild, recent-onset psoriasis with methotrexate.

Case 5C. The same patient presented in Case 5B made the same request, but on this occasion was in her first trimester of pregnancy. Methotrexate is teratogenic and therefore contraindicated in pregnant women.

Cases and Their Analysis

Case 1 (Demand for Disability) and Case 2 (Demand for Hospitalization)

These two cases involve the physician in the role of societally licensed technician who is expert in deciding on the appropriate utilization of limited societal resources—in these cases, disability payments or hospitalization. This role of the physician has sometimes been referred to as the "gatekeeper" role.[1] Although the government and private insurance companies have developed guidelines (eligibility criteria) that must be met to qualify for these benefits, there remains considerable room for discretionary

[1]Deborah A. Stone, "Physicians as Gatekeepers: Illness Certification as a Rationing Device," *Public Policy*, XXVII (spring, 1979), 227–54.

judgment in individual cases. The physician is expected to apply the standards established by the insurer in as just a manner as possible, giving each individual his or her due. Once a physician has applied appropriate standards and procedures and concludes that a particular patient does not qualify for a given benefit, he or she has made a technical-value decision in the role of societal agent. As with all other medical decisions, these allocational decisions are made in the face of uncertainty and thus are subject to error. Furthermore, the need to make such decisions may place the physician in the uncomfortable position of wanting to provide maximum benefits for each patient while being prevented from doing so by the rules, regulations, and laws governing the allocation of particular benefits. The fact that a physician is in a position to make this type of allocational judgment is a function of the physician role. However, the standards that must be employed in reaching the decision apply to the physician not only in the role as physician but also in the role of moral agent. In both cases 1 and 2, the physician is encouraged to lie (commit perjury) and act fradulently. It should be clear that the physician is not obliged to act immorally or illegally simply to satisfy a particular patient demand.

Case 3 (Demand for a CAT Scan)

In this case, the physician is functioning as expert technician but is again serving a function as a licensed gatekeeper of medicine's technological resources. There is also a power struggle going on between the patient and the physician regarding which is the "expert" capable of assessing the severity and significance of symptoms and of deciding whether a given diagnostic procedure is necessary or appropriate. The patient might claim that her privileged knowledge of the states of her own body merits attention comparable to the physician's belief that a CAT scan is unnecessary. These scans are expensive and are a relatively limited technological resource, but most scanning machines are not utilized to their full capacity. Although the physician as physician and the physician as citizen bears some responsibility for controlling the costs of medical care, economic considerations are not paramount in this case. Rather, the power struggle revolves around who has the knowledge and power (or perhaps who *ought* to have the power) to order or to refuse to order the procedure. The physician's decision was based primarily on the feeling that the test was unnecessary and medically inappropriate and that ordering and reordering CAT scans constituted bad and inappropriate medicine.

Case 4 (Demand for Sleeping Pills)

The physician's refusal to agree to the patient's demands in this case were based on several considerations:

1. The major reason for refusing the patient's demand was the potential risk to the patient. The combination of alcohol and sleeping pills is dangerous in general and increases the potential for suicide or inadvertent drug interactions in susceptible patients. Most sleeping pills are long-acting; they also interact with alcohol and might impair the patient's ability to drive her car each morning. Thus, treating her with sleeping pills while knowing that she consumed large quantities of alcohol might pose risks for the patient's own health and would constitute poor medical practice.

2. Sleeping pills were perceived to be an inappropriate therapy in this case. The patient's insomnia appeared to be symptomatic of an underlying severe depression. The suppression of the symptom, sleeplessness, was the

"treatment" demanded by the patient. The physician preferred to encourage the patient to do something specifically for the cause of the symptom, the depression.

3. The demanded treatment would probably have been ineffective. A recent article notes, "The beneficial effect, if
any, of a hypnotic drug upon sleep is typically to reduce
the time needed to fall asleep by 10–20 minutes and to
lengthen the night's total sleep time by 20–40 minutes.
The importance of these effects is unclear at present."[2]
Even if hypnotic drugs are temporarily effective, their
effectiveness ceases in a short time.

4. This treatment involves risks to others by compromising
the patient's ability to drive an automobile. No reliable
data exist on the relationship between the use of hypnotic
drugs (particularly when combined with alcohol) and traffic
accidents or fatalities, although there is a strong suspicion
that there is such a relationship.

5. The physician felt uneasy about regarding insomnia as a
medical problem. The question also arose whether physicians (at least, physicians other than psychiatrists) could
or should manage it.

Cases 5, 5A, 5B, and 5C (Demand for Dangerous Treatment)

In this series of cases there is another power struggle between patient and physician, but in these instances the notion
of imminent danger to the patient becomes more important. In
the previous case of the alcoholic professor, the potential risks
of the treatment were statistical and were projected into the
future. In these cases, however, the risks to the patient are im-

---

[2]Frederic Solomon et al., "Sleeping Pills, Insomnia and Medical Practice," New
England Journal of Medicine, CCC (April 1979), 803–08.

mediate and direct. The angiogram is not an indicated medical procedure under the circumstances. It is inappropriate and unnecessary; an angiogram is an invasive procedure and dangerous (although the danger of death in a healthy patient is low). One might agree to perform the electrocardiogram and the exercise test—even though they might not have been necessary—in part because they imparted no risk to the patient. But the conscientious physician would refuse to order a more risky study such as the coronary angiogram. One further point is that in these situations the risk to the patient arises as a result of the diagnostic study or treatment which the physician is being asked to provide; thus, the action of the physician is related directly to the risk for the patient.

Case 5A. Once again, the risk in this situation must be taken into account. If the patient's liver disease worsens, it may become irreversible. There is also a question of whether the patient's obesity warrants these extreme risks. Finally, there is a lingering doubt about whether obesity (exogenous type) is a medical problem.

Cases 5B and 5C. Again, there is a potential for causing irreversible harm (particularly to the fetus) by treating with methotrexate. Note here that the physician refuses to use medical arts in such a way that the medical action will likely cause harm to another, in this case the fetus. Further, it appears that the extreme treatment is not warranted in either Case 5B or 5C because the patient has only a mild case of psoriasis.

A Description of Patient Demands

The Cause of Patient Demands

Many factors have contributed to changes in the physician–patient relationship and to the emergence of this new class of

demanding patients. These factors include (1) a change in the
nature of medicine transforming it from an empiric art into a
scientific, specialized discipline involving a massive bureaucracy;
(2) the emergence of "rights" language and consumerism, and a
change in attitudes in society toward all professionals including
physicians; (3) the removal of economic restraints on health services by the development of various entitlement programs, extensive third-party health insurance programs, and the establishment of organizations offering prepaid medical care. Another
factor that is often not emphasized is the role physicians and
medicine have played in contributing to patient demands. They
have done so by overselling the achievements of medicine; urging
on the public certain tests or treatments which have not been
proved efficacious; participating passively or actively in permitting the boundaries of medicine to expand to include many social,
behavioral, and criminal problems that were not considered medical in the past; pursuing their own economic self-interest by
sometimes encouraging marginally unnecessary surgery, office
visits, diagnostic studies, and procedures. Thus, many factors
related to physicians, patients, economics, and general societal
trends have been involved in the emergence of this new group
of demanding patients.

What Is a Patient Demand?[3]

A demand in medicine is a statement by which a patient
claims from a physician (or other health professional), as an entitlement, a specific medical service that the patient believes is
both a medical service and one which physicians ought to provide.
Thus, the patient not only indicates the goals he or she is pursuing

[3]Jerry Avorn, "Needs, Demands, and Interests: Their Intersection in Health Care
  Delivery," Chapter 7, in this volume.

in visiting a physician (an entirely appropriate and necessary part of the medical encounter) but specifies the particular means by which the goal will be achieved. The patient presents not only with a complaint but with a demand for a specific means to redress the complaint. One might say that a demand in medicine is a situation in which the patient tells the doctor exactly what he or she wants from medicine—not in general terms, but with great specificity. [4] Medical demands are often phrased in the language of "rights"; they are advanced in an adversarial and contentious fashion.

What Is a Demanding Patient? [5]

Demanding patient often share one or several of the following characteristics:

1. Their style tends to disturb the decorum of standard physician–patient interactions in which the relationship between the parties is often physician-controlled or mutual. These demanding patients invert the traditional model and would make the physician a passive agent who is required to practice under the direction and control of the patient.
2. Demanding patients attempt to short-circuit a traditional function of the physician, which is to decide whether a particular patient's complaint is truly a medical one and one that ought to be managed within the medical context.
3. Demanding patients demand not only a service but a particular, specified service. Normally, a physician uti-

---

[4] Arthur L. Caplan, "How Should Values Count in the Allocation of New Technologies in Health Care," Chapter 4, in this volume.
[5] Eliot Friedson, "Prepaid Group Practice and the New 'Demanding Patient,' " *Milbank Memorial Fund Quarterly*, (Fall, 1973), 473–88.

lizes his or her medical knowledge and clinical judgment
to propose to a patient a plan of treatment, alternatives
to the plan, and the relative risks and benefits of each
possibility. The demanding patient, however, specifies a
service that may or may not be medically correct or even
feasible. Such patients may deny that the physician's expertise has any relevance except insofar as the physician's
decisions coincide with their own desires.

Obligations of the Individual Physician to Demanding Patients

Beginning with the cases in which patient demands were
rejected, I find it worthwhile to describe the reasons for such
actions. Clinical situations arise in which the physician would and
should refuse to honor the demands of a competent patient. This
refusal would be based upon the physician's role as a discerning
moral agent and a discerning physician. The physician would be
uneasy, uncomfortable, and dissatisfied in acquiescing to a patient's demands in such cases. Such a physician would feel badly
as a person and would feel that his or her behavior was inappropriate to the circumstances, sensing that the proposed actions would be unprofessional and not consonant with the physician role. The cases presented are examples of some of the
situations in which physicians did not and should not comply with
patient demands.

Within limits to be specified later, refusal to honor patients
demands in cases such as those described should be general and
should, in principle, be expected of all physicians. This implies
a normative claim about what medicine should be like. Such

refusals, it is claimed, should be made by most physicians in their roles as physicians. This normative notion of what it is to be a physician should guide physicians' decisions in a large number of cases. This implies a vision of medicine as a profession that should have a high degree of articulate self-definition.

A few disclaimers and limits are appropriate regarding this normative claim.

Disclaimers

No empirical claim is being made that all or even most physicians would act in precisely the way indicated. Many competent physicians—perhaps most—would, but this is a normative discussion and not a summary of empirical observations.

Obviously, not all physicians are equally competent technically and, in individual circumstances, a particular physician may be wrong and the patient may be correct in demanding a particular treatment. Yet in such cases, the physician ought to act in accordance with his or her sincere belief about what the appropriate and fitting course of action should be.

Naturally, the practice of physician shopping exists: a demanded treatment or test—even one that may pose a risk for the patient—can almost always be obtained from some physician or surgeon, particularly if payment is assured. This unfortunate circumstance is encouraged in principle by some advocates of a libertarian model of medicine in which health care is seen as a product to be provided by physician-technicians and consumed by patient-clients. The fact that a physician or surgeon can be found who will acquiesce to almost any demand does not negate the normative claim that such behavior is unfitting and inappropriate in medicine.

Limits

The generalized argument that on occasion physicians should decide to refuse patient demands must be understood within limits. Some of these limits are the following:

Medical decisions are always made with varying degrees of uncertainty. Any particular decision may turn out to be wrong. Therefore, other equally competent, equally scrupulous physicians with identical value systems might, on the basis of technical and clinical considerations, reach different decisions regarding cases. This fact does not negate the claim that in principle such decisions are generalizable. It merely suggests that in medicine there is always room for clinical disagreement on technical grounds.

In reaching any decision (for example, to provide or refuse to provide the demanded service), there always remains the psychological difficulty of being clear about the motivations of oneself or others. There is often a fine line in such decisions between rationalization and reason giving.

There exist classes of physicians (e.g., Catholic, Marxist, or libertarian physicians) who operate with a systematic set of values not embraced entirely by the profession or by the society. Such physicians may, as a group, make decisions that are fairly uniform among themselves but are not typical of the profession as a whole. For example, a libertarian physician might respond to any request a rational patient could pay for, or a Catholic physician might refuse to perform abortions except in circumstances where the mother's life was directly threatened, and sometimes not even then. In such instances, the private values of the physician would dictate his or her responses to a particular patient's demands. Despite the reality of such value differences among certain subsets of physicians, the profession of medicine has probably not evolved radically divergent views of its proper role and self-definition. This reality of value differences modifies and delimits but does not negate the normative claim that some expectations are generalizable in the practice of medicine and that there should be agreement among physicians regarding proper professional behavior in a wide range of cases.

Obligations of the Medical Profession to Demanding Patients

Thus far, it has been suggested that in certain situations a physician should not accede to some medical demands of a rational patient. A normative claim was made, so far undefended, that physicians as a professional group, within the limits of technical disagreements, should generally refuse to accede to certain demands made by rational patients. What practical consequences might this normative principle of generalizability have for medicine?

If, for the moment, the correctness of the normative claim is granted—that is, if situations exist in which physicians generally should refuse to satisfy specific patient demands—what options would then exist for applying this principle to specific cases? If one thinks about how this might work in practice, two extreme general lines appear: (1) one might weigh the concern for consistency most heavily and advocate institutionalization of the principles and attempt to ensure their uniform application or (2) one might encourage the individual judgment of physicians while hoping for some emerging professional uniformity. In the latter instance, one would then disseminate the principles, seek professional agreement on them, and then allow them to be applied on a discretionary basis by individual physicians. Neither solution in its pure form is entirely satisfying. Nevertheless, it is useful for purposes of clarity to examine the implications of each in isolation and to explore their positive and negative features.

Institutionalization of Ways to Respond to Patient Demands

If one weighs heavily the preference for consistency, one might attempt to institutionalize the generalizable principles. This might involve developing a set of standard procedures to be followed in all cases of a particular kind and would be one way to achieve consistency and uniformity. Such an approach might weed out serious errors and perhaps even detect and eliminate unscrupulous, fraudulent, or incompetent physicians who can currently manipulate a system that lacks clear-cut institutional rules. This system would also permit patients and society to know the procedures by which such decisions are made and to have a formal system for seeking redress of unfavorable decisions.

The following arguments might be raised against institutionalizing such principles: New administrative structures and an expanded bureaucracy (which would inevitably introduce its own irrationalities) might be required to apply these principles to patient demands. Formal rules are rarely flexible enough to conform to the particularity of individual cases. Such institutionalization would immediately limit the discretion of individual physicians and severely compromise the sanctity of the patient–physician relationship. If required second opinions before elective surgery are viewed as a mild example of such institutional rules, one could imagine the establishment of committees to review all major nonemergency decisions in advance. Team medicine as practiced in large medical centers offers one example of decision making by committees composed primarily of professionals. The ultimate extension of this bureaucratic maneuver might generate a system in which individual physicians could make decisions only if they conformed fully to the established and institutionalized norms of the profession.

Encourage Individual Decisions by Physicians as a Way to Respond to Patient Demands

Consider the opposite argument. Even if there were general agreement on the correctness of the generalizable principles, arguments against institutionalizing them could be offered. Rather, one might wish to encourage the primacy of individual physician judgment. The arguments here are those traditional to medicine and to the medical model. In this situation, the highest value to be defended is the integrity of the patient–physician relationship and the freedom of individual patients and physicians to reach proper decisions in individual cases. This may be a better solution than a bureaucratic structure that would surely become complex and authoritarian. On utilitarian grounds, it may be better to allow many doctors and patients to make various choices in order that the best solution may finally be found; it may prove to be better than a generalizable, bureaucratic solution. Of course, if these principles were shared by the medical community, they could serve as medical ideals even if they were not formally institutionalized. Such ideals might serve as a standard; even if they were not enforceable by law, they might be enforceable by custom or by professional code obligations.

There are, however, arguments against encouraging the primacy of individual physician judgment: such a system might reinforce the radical pluralism of physicians' judgment and would probably tend to support a paternalistic model of medicine. The physician's role as father, priest, scientist, and individual entrepreneur would be enhanced. Thus, the failure to institutionalize generalizable principles might leave one with principles that were nothing more than rhetoric.

Exploration of Medical Discernment

This paper has suggested that a physician might refuse to honor certain demands made by competent patients. That claim quickly generates a sense of unease. Is it appropriate for physicians to frustrate the demands of rational individuals who consider themselves to be in a doctor–patient relationship? This discussion continues by exploring more deeply some of the reasons and motives that might lead a physician to discern that patient demands should be refused, as in the case examples previously presented. Before attempting to draw out the relevant factors involved in medical discernment in the specific cases presented, a few words about the term *discernment* are in order.

I am persuaded that thinking about actual cases in medicine follows a pattern similar to that described by James Gustafson in his essay on moral discernment in the Christian life,[6] rather than a conceptually simpler, but probably for that very reason false, procedural checklist for making moral–technical decisions. As Gustafson indicates, the nature of moral discernment is more analogous to esthetic judgment than to mathematical analysis; therefore even subtle variations in these complex cases could cause a change of opinion. Gustafson's complex essay defies simple summary, but at one point in his argument he states:

> The discerning act of moral discernment is impossible to program and difficult to describe. It involves perceptivity, discrimination, subtlety, sensitivity, clarity, rationality, and accuracy. And while some men seem to have it as a "gift of the gods," others achieve it by experience and training, by learning and acting.[7]

---

[6]James M. Gustafson, "Moral Discernment in the Christian Life," in *Theology and Christian Ethics,* edited by James M. Gustafson, (Philadelphia: United Church Press,), pp. 99–119.
[7]Ibid., p. 109.

The most important feature of this model of medical discernment is precisely that an exhaustive, rational explanation—let alone a detailed description of mental processes—is impossible, but that an approximation of it nevertheless presents a much more accurate picture of the way medical judgments are made than any conceptually neater pattern can.

It must never be forgotten that the physician's relationship to the patient is premised on specific technical training and competency. This specialized knowledge and proficiency is utilized to assist patients in curing or ameliorating their illness and disease and in overcoming the fear, pain, and suffering that are often associated with ill health. Once sought out by the patient, the physician becomes involved in the patient's problem. The physician is personally accountable to the patient if he or she fails to perform the task adequately because of lack of skill or negligence or because, for whatever reason, the physician fails to act in the patient's behalf. The intensity and particularity of medical situations demand fitting and appropriate responses from physicians, and such decisions are based upon medical discernment.

Medical discernment is a product of (1) the physician's specialized knowledge and clinical wisdom as a physician, (2) the goals and ideals of the medical profession and society as they are interpreted by a particular physician, and (3) the qualities (i.e., perceptivity, sensitivity, clarity, etc.) of the individual physician as an individual decision maker. In different circumstances, one or another of these elements in decision making may predominate. In general, however, decisions are reached on the basis of the consideration and assessment of each of these factors. Specifically, the claim is not being advanced that physicians as physicians possess a unique or special moral sense that always leads to a discerning decision. Rather, the individual physician's knowledge about the technical aspects of medicine and about the ideals of the medical profession, along with the basic personality of the physician, should combine to lead to a discerning choice. However, in individual cases inadequate technical knowledge and insufficient understanding of the ideals of the medical profession or personal failures may result in a poor, nondiscerning decision.

The process of discernment is analogous in many ways to traditional clinical judgment and must be contrasted with alternative approaches such as the application of moral principles. In the latter approach, one attempts to determine a morally correct decision by formally applying general moral considerations such as rules, principles, and laws. After beginning with the general moral consideration, one strives to determine whether the general consideration arises in particular cases, and if it does, how the rule or principle is to be applied to determine a proper course of action.

By contrast, discernment involves the ability to draw relevant distinctions, to discard extraneous facts, to penetrate to the heart of the matter, and to make choices of one course of action as the better among many possible ones. That choice can be defended as "better" not in some absolute sense but because, given the available facts and their interpretation, judicious reflection suggests that it fits the actual situation more adequately than other available options.[8-10]

Of course, a discerning decision is based upon an appeal to some system of belief, rules, or moral principles. Right choices about how to provide patients with good medical care require this medical discernment. Gustafson's comments on the "dis-

[8]Stephen Toulmin, "The Tyranny of Principles," Hastings Center Report, XI (December, 1981), 31–39.

[9]Arthur L. Caplan, "Ethical Engineers Need Not Apply: The States of Applied Ethics Today," Science, Technology, and Human Values, VI (fall, 1980), 24–32.

[10]Arthur L. Caplan, "Applying Morality to Advances in Biomedicine: Can and Should This Be Done?" New Knowledge in the Biomedical Sciences, edited by W. Bondeson et al. (Dordrecht, Holland: Reidel, 1982), pp. 155–68.

cerning moral man" can be applied to the discerning medical practitioner:

> He can think clearly about potential consequences and applicable principles; he knows something about the range of values that might compete with or support each other, and he can discriminate between alternative courses of action. He is likely to have a clear head, to be able to argue with himself and others before a judgment is made, and give good reasons for it afterward.[11]

To conclude: a physician might utilize medical discernment to determine that in a particular set of circumstances the most appropriate and right action is to refuse the demands made by a patient.

General Reasons Why a Physician Should Sometimes Reject Patient Demands

A physician might sometimes reject a patient demand on the basis of

1. General moral principles that apply to physicians and to all moral agents
2. Uncertainty concerning the limits of one's role and responsibility as a physician
3. Responsibilities in one's role as a good physician

Refusals Based on General Moral Principles Applicable to All Moral Agents and Therefore to Physicians

Although the specific medical demands made of the physician can only be made to one in the role of physician, the reason for some refusals may not be role-related. Refusal can be justified

---

[11]Gustafson, "Moral Discernment," pp. 108–9.

if one is asked to commit an immoral act such as lying, breaking promises, doing evil, acting unjustly, or breaking the morally valid laws of a civil society. These moral principles should not, in general, be violated even for the sake of the patient's benefit (e.g., hospitalization for a patient who has hospital insurance or disability payments and more extensive medical care for a hard-working widow with chronic disease). In such instances, the physician can exercise medical discernment and refuse to accede to the patient's demands. Alternatively, in particular instances, the physician's discernment might dictate a decision to acquiesce in the patient's demand even when doing so might involve engaging in an illegal act. For the physician, this would be a form of civil disobedience and would require public announcement, justification, and the willingness to bear the consequences of the action.

Refusals May Be Based on Uncertainty Concerning the Limits of One's Role and Responsibility as a Physician

Refusals may be based neither on role definition nor on general moral principles but precisely on uncertainty concerning the extent and limit of one's role and responsibilities. A physician may be uncertain whether a particular demand made by a patient is one that is appropriate for physicians to respond to in their role as physicians. For example, the following situation is one in which most morally conscientious people could agree on the physician's responsibility as physician. Consider the case of a poor man who came to a physician's office complaining of hunger. The physician noted that the man was malnourished and cachectic. The man demanded that the doctor give him $20 so that he could buy food. A doctor could legitimately refuse to honor this demand on the ground that it fell outside of proper medical responsibilities, even though as a person he or she might have a responsibility to offer help to a neighbor; or the physician might decide to honor the demand of the person (note: not "the patient") on the grounds of charity. The man's request would not have been made legitimately to the physician in the role of physician.

Perhaps the weakness of the example just cited is the apparent clarity of the circumstances. Poverty has not yet been defined as a medical disease. One appropriate response to the individual's request would be to refer him to some other societal institution such as a state welfare agency, a church, or a philanthropic organization whose role it is to attend to the needs of the poor.

Unfortunately, the proper institutional jurisdiction for many human problems is less clear cut than for poverty, either because the problems resemble medical issues or because alternate societal institutions have abnegated their responsibilities. Such difficult problems as alcoholism, neurotic anxiety and depression, unhappiness, unattractiveness, aging, exogenous obesity, nonorganic sexual dysfunction, accident proneness, smoking, and "sports medicine" have all come to be regarded by some as within the medical sphere. Thus, when patients make certain demands of physicians, there is often considerable lack of clarity about whether such demands are appropriately made to medical personnel or institutions. Perhaps one role of the physician is to utilize expert technical knowledge of, for example, the physiology of obesity or alcoholism to assist society in determining whether obesity or alcoholism are properly medical problems. Even if alcohol is declared a medical and not a police problem (this is a societal determination), physicians caring for poor, uneducated, unemployed, relationless chronic alcoholics suffering from recurring medical complications of alcoholism may remain unclear as to whether their responsibilities to such individuals extend beyond management of recurring medical complications.

The Responsibilities of the Good Physician

The final general ground for a physician's refusal of a patient's demand is based on his or her responsibilities in the role of good physician as determined by societal expectations, professional standards, and individual standards.

One perspective from which to examine the role of the physician is that of the societally defined institution of medicine and its relationship to other institutions of society, especially as those are manifest in the administrative functions of the physician. In these instances, the physician's medical judgment is a necessary condition for some other purpose of societal function. In this regard, the physician has obligations not only to his patients but also to the broader society. These obligations are derived in part from custom, but many of them have become formalized through legal requirements. For example, the physician has a duty to report patients with certain contagious diseases to public health authorities and to report patients who are clearly a danger to themselves or others to police authorities. Further, during the past 150 years, as society has increasingly licensed physicians and as the bureaucracy of both medicine and government has increased, physicians have come to fill a role as agent and administrator for society. It is the physician's responsibility to complete insurance forms and disability forms and to determine the medical suitability of pilots, military personnel, and—in some instances— even drivers of automobiles. In the situations cited, the physician determines that certain persons are suitable according to legally established criteria to perform such functions. These types of cases involve some matters of judgment. The criteria established by government agencies are not so precise as to eliminate all judgment calls, but the range of judgment required of the physician is clearly constricted.

In contrast to these tasks, which are explicit administrative responsibilities of the physician and can only be performed legally by a physician, there is still another level at which the physician functions as a societal agent. The physician serves a gatekeeper function for society,[12] admitting people to aspects of the medical system in accordance with his or her best medical judgment. This type of judgment is based upon the physician's "medical discernment." The physician is the one who has been charged to determine whether a patient requires hospitalization or whether certain procedures are indicated in individual circumstances. He or she has been licensed to prescribe "ethical" drugs and such medications are not legally available except by prescription. These cases involve criteria that are less explicit than in the category of administrative responsibilities. They require that the physician conform to the highest standards of medical practice and require a high degree of individual judgment on the part of physicians.

It is not the physician's obligation to make basic judgments about allocational questions. These must be determined by the broader institutions of society. But at the level of the individual patient, the physician has the task of determining whether an individual patient will receive a particular drug, test, or operation or will be hospitalized. It is therefore the physician's obligation to administer these functions prudently and not frivolously, and to do so in accordance with the best medical judgment.

In addition to refusing patients' demands based on their societal role, physicians might refuse patients' demand on the basis of their self-defined roles as "good" physicians. The traits that which are involved in being a good physician are difficult to

[12]Robert M. Veatch, "Professional Medical Ethics: The Grounding of Its Principles," *Journal of Medicine & Philosophy*, IV (1979), 1–19.

define and even more difficult to justify, but they nevertheless exist. We would think badly of a physician who treated tension headaches with morphine, or painful, chronic rheumatoid arthritis with high doses of corticosteroids. Although in both instances the symptoms would be suppressed, our criticism of the physician would be based on his or her poor judgment in selecting unnecessarily powerful drugs and drugs that result in unacceptable risks. And our opinion of the physician would not change, even if we later learned that each of these treatments was a treatment demanded by the patient or that each was paid for by the patient. On the one hand, knowing the treatment was demanded might permit us to think more positively about the technical knowledge of the physician; it might serve to mitigate our charge of gross incompetence or even of negligence, unscrupulousness, or fraud. But our knowledge that the physician was persuaded by a demanding patient to act in ways that could permanently alter or harm the patient—that the patient urged and abetted the physician to act in ways counter to the physician's own concept of good medical practice—might lead us to be even more harsh in our moral indictment of the physician. It was not the practitioner's technical knowledge that was deficient but rather his or her character; being a weak and manipulable individual, the physician lacked "medical discernment."

In my estimation, the "good" physician is one who acts in a manner appropriate to the particular patient's medical problem and who does so while maintaining personal integrity and conscientiousness. We should not discount the possibility that the physician can make mistakes, but even when one is technically wrong about a matter, one is morally obliged to act in accordance with the dictates of medical discernment. In determining how to act appropriately regarding the demanding patient, the physician assesses the potential benefits and the potential harm of a particular diagnostic or therapeutic maneuver which a patient had demanded. As the potential for harm increases and as the likelihood of benefit diminishes, the physician's determination to resist a particular demand should increase. If the potential for harm is a virtual certainty and the chance for benefit negligible, the physician would be derelict in yielding to the demand. This is definitely the case when the harm that might result from the intervention is irreversible or immediately life-threatening. In addition to the risk and essential irreversibility involved in such cases, the physician who strives to act appropriately would also determine whether a particular procedure were necessary or unnecessary. Thus, even if procedures like a CAT scan are not risky, they may be unnecessary and thus inappropriate. Finally, the physician may take account of the cost of the procedure. Cost-consciousness at the level of the individual physician should be taken into account, but only if it coincides with or reinforces one or more of the previously stated criteria of appropriateness.

Conclusion

The point of view regarding medical discernment discussed here has been criticized by many writers in recent years, perhaps most persistently by Robert Veatch. In a recent essay on professional medical ethics,[13] Veatch argues that the foundation of medical ethics is a triple contract: (1) a basic social contract, (2) a contract between the profession and society, and (3) a third contract between individual doctors or groups of doctors and individual patients or groups of patients. Veatch would permit, perhaps even encourage, considerable latitude and discretion in this third contract as long as the decisions were mutually agreed upon by doctor and patient and were not unilaterally imposed by physicians. Presumably, this third contract between individual phy-

[13]Ibid.

sicians and patients takes account of peculiar value-laden orientations, such as might be found, for example, in certain Catholic
or libertarian physicians or in certain Catholic or libertarian patients. If patients were informed of the value stance of their
physicians and physicians were informed of such value stances of
their patients, both could voluntarily elect to enter or not to enter
into this third contract. Thus, based upon the voluntariness and
mutuality of this third contract, Veatch would presumably agree
that a patient's particular demand might be refused on the basis
of the specifications of this third contract.

Veatch's notion of the second contract, a contract between
the profession and society, is more difficult. He notes that professional codes or oaths

> merely express a sense of mutual obligation among professionals,
> but society should not accept such agreements as binding on society
> whenever they impact outside the profession. If the professionals
> had agreed among themselves that the physician's duty is to do
> what he thinks will benefit the patient or to do no harm to the
> patient, or even to do what professional groups believe is in the
> public interest, it still must remain an open question whether so-
> ciety concurs that such a principle is reasonable for governing re-
> lationships with members of a society.[14]

Thus, in Veatch's terms, the contract between the professional and society ought to be a mutual agreement. In this regard,
the observations regarding cases above can be viewed as an effort
to describe certain positions or values to which physicians should
subscribe. If the second contract between the profession and
society is dyadic, one may understand those values as suggesting
some of the bargaining positions from which physicians might
begin their negotiations with the larger society. Of course, "society" (in practice, government) might finally choose to overrule
those perceptions of the proper responses of the profession and
of professionals to some patient demands. Whether this would
be a prudent course is a question for further consideration.

[14]Ibid., p. 15.

ACKNOWLEDGMENTS

I am indebted to Professor Martin Cook of Santa Clara University for his suggestions and critical comments on earlier drafts of this essay.

Appendix A

List of Essential and Important Health Standards for Prison Health Care

Section A.   ADMINISTRATIVE

Section B.   PERSONNEL

122   Licensure (Essential)
123   Job Descriptions (Essential)
124   Staff Development and Training
125   Professional Publications
126   Health Appraisal Personnel (Essential)
127   Medications Administration Training (Essential)
128   Training for Emergency Situations (Essential)
129   First Aid Training
130   Training of Staff Regarding Mental Illness and Chemical
              Dependency (Essential)
131   Health and Hygiene Requirements: Food Service
              Workers
132   Utilization of Volunteers
133   Inmate Workers (Essential)

Section C.   CARE AND TREATMENT

134   Levels of Care
135   Treatment Philosophy
136   Continuity of Care
137   Access to Treatment (Essential)
138   Direct Orders (Essential)
139   Standing Orders
140   Receiving Screening (Essential)
141   Delousing
142   Health Appraisals (Essential)
143   Dental Care
144   Interim Health Appraisals: Mentally ill and Retarded
145   Daily Triaging of Complaints (Essential)
146   Sick Call (Essential)
147   Health Evaluations: Inmates in Isolation
148   Chemically Dependent Inmates
149   Detoxification (Essential)
150   Special Medical Program
151   Infirmary Care (Essential)
152   Hospital Care
153   Preventive Care
154   Emergency Services (Essential)
155   Chronic and Convalescent Care
156   Pregnant Inmates
157   Nutritional Requirements

Index